Just Two More Bites!

Just Two More Bites!

HELPING PICKY EATERS
SAY YES TO FOOD

LINDA PIETTE, MS, RD

THREE RIVERS PRESS • NEW YORK

The stories in this book represent fictionalized composites of children and families the author has worked with over a twenty-five-year period. None of the names in this book refers to an actual child or family member.

Grateful acknowledgment is made to the following for permission to reprint previously published material: **The Food Allergy & Anaphylaxis Network:** "How to Read a Label for a Milk-Free Diet," "How to Read a Label for an Egg-Free Diet," and "How to Read a Label for a Peanut-Free Diet." Copyright © by The Food Allergy Network. **The University of Minnesota:** Figure showing changes in body growth, keeping height constant, adapted from *The Development of the External Dimensions of the Human Body in the Fetal Period* by Richard E. Scammon and Leroy A. Calkins. Copyright © 1929 by the University of Minnesota. Reprinted by permission of the University of Minnesota. **Marci Campbell and Kristine Kelsey:** The Peach Survey by Marci Campbell and Kristine Kelsey, as published in the *Journal of the American Dietic Association,* October 1994. Reprinted by permission of Marci Campbell and Kristine Kelsey.

Published in the United States by Three Rivers Press, an imprint of the Crown Publishing Group, a division of Random House, Inc., New York.
www.crownpublishing.com
Three Rivers Press and the Tugboat design are registered trademarks of Random House, Inc.

Library of Congress Cataloging-in-Publication Data
Piette, Linda D.
Just two more bites!: helping picky eaters say "yes" to food/Linda D. Piette.
Includes bibliographical references.
1. Food preferences in children.   2. Children—Nutrition.
3. Children—Nutrition—Psychological aspects.   4. Child rearing.   I. Title.
HQ784.E3P54 2006
649'.3—dc22   2006007810
ISBN-10: 1-4000-8109-2
ISBN-13: 978-1-4000-8109-7

Printed in the United States of America
Design by Helene Berinsky
10 9 8 7 6 5 4 3 2 1
First Edition

CONTENTS

ACKNOWLEDGMENTS

Writing a book is a big undertaking and one I could not have accomplished without the help and support of others. I thank my husband, Don, for his steadfast encouragement; my agent, Judith Riven, for her faith, responsiveness, and advice; the families and staff from the Professional Center and Cambridge Head Start for their stories and insights.

For helping me write more clearly, I thank my editors, Kathryn McHugh and Lindsey Moore, and the three special women in my writers' group: Joan Cass, Deb Hagan, and Sarah Auerbach.

For their encouragement and feedback, I thank Dr. Alan Crocker, Beth Horning, Dr. Ronald E. Klienman, Dr. Deb Turiano, Dr. Allan Rosenberg, June Piette, and Joanna Bond.

For favors big and small I thank Maria Bartlett, Cynthia Bayerl, Nancy Clark, Sherry Cohen, Molly Holland, Fran Peterson, Rena Prendergast, Gino Zaccardelli, and Helena Szudy.

And last, I thank my parents, Anna and Rinaldo DiCocco, for giving me love, good food, and the inspiration to dream.

INTRODUCTION

Is your child's picky eating a passing stage or something more? For years, pediatricians and well-meaning relatives have told parents not to fret over a young child's food refusals, identifying picky eating as just a stage that most children outgrow. But many parents, struggling to provide their kids with a reasonable, nutritious diet, find this advice too dismissive.

They may be onto something. Proof abounds that millions of kids are not outgrowing their early pickiness. According to the Healthy Eating Index (HEI), developed by the Center for Nutrition Policy and Promotion of the U.S. Department of Agriculture, 70 percent of American children have diets defined as "needing improvement." The scores actually get worse as children grow older.

It's true that toddlers are notorious for refusing food. Age and developmental stages play a key role in when and why children say no to food. But new issues are also emerging. Parents with their own food or diet concerns, busier lifestyles, and advances in medical technology add new complexities. For a small but growing number of children, food refusals are longer-lasting and more deep-rooted. Many children are at risk for feeding disorders. Babies born early, and those with autism or other special needs, often struggle with eating. A surprisingly high number of children under age five fall into one of these categories.

- According to the October 2002 issue of *Pediatric News,* 25 percent of young children have some form of feeding disorder. The number increases to more than 50 percent in autistic children and to 80 percent in children with developmental delays.

Furthermore, the number of such children is growing:

- According to government figures, the number of children with a low birth weight has increased slowly but steadily since 1984.
- The number of special needs children in public schools has risen over the last twenty years. Since 1986, with the passage of legislation mandating early intervention services nationally, the number of children receiving services has grown steadily.

While more and more children have these medical and biological conditions, they are also more likely to have parents or siblings with their own food issues.

Family members with their own food struggles are less equipped to help and may actually compound a young child's eating problems. Researchers from Stanford University found differences in how mothers with past or present eating disorders presented food to their children. As Americans face an epidemic rise in obesity and other eating disorders, parents and other family members are likely to be even more concerned when a young child refuses food. Many want ideas on how to cope better with these challenges.

Eating problems can be complex, emotionally charged, and difficult to solve. To make matters worse, children grow and change from one day to the next, so it's sometimes hard to determine where one problem ends and another begins. In order to cope with your picky eater, it's necessary to recognize the multiple influences of your child's developmental stage, social dynamics, nutrition, sensory issues, and feeding skills. Collaborative work with other health professionals has helped me to see picky eaters in a broader context. I have watched speech therapists help children with chewing and swallowing, physical and occupational therapists help children with sensory issues or motor skills, and social workers and psychologists provide helpful insights into social dynamics.

The reasons why kids refuse food can be nonsensical and, at times, maddening. It is easy to lose perspective. *Just Two More Bites!* (that familiar refrain) explores ways to make eating more enjoyable for children. But there are limits to what you can do, and it is important to recognize those limits. This book will show you the situations in which you can influence your child's eating for the better. It also explores situations in which picky eating is more than a passing phase and lists resources to help you find specialized help, if need be.

You won't find magical recipes guaranteed to make your child eat. But you will find

- Guidelines on how to recognize whether picky eating is a health problem for your child
- Real-life answers about how to handle day-to-day food struggles
- Tips for finding and filling nutrition gaps
- Strategies for children with heightened sensitivities to food textures or flavors
- Information about "feeding specialists" and other resources

Over the last twenty-five years, I have worked as a pediatric nutritionist and registered dietitian in early intervention, preschool programs, and private and public schools. During that time, I have observed more than one thousand picky eaters and listened to their parents. I have watched my young clients and learned from their struggles. In a sense, their stories have become my stories, and I use them to illustrate what I have learned about picky eaters in the pages of this book.

I hope that the stories of other children combined with practical tips and research findings by social scientists give you insight and inspiration to improve mealtimes for you and your family.

PART

I

Solving the Puzzle of Picky Eating

Ralph and Katy Greene are committed to having family meals. They juggle work, long commutes, music lessons, and nap times so that they can share at least one meal a day with their three kids. Yet family mealtimes are not working out as planned.

Instead of warm, bonding experiences, they are nonstop battles. No matter what the food, the kids whine and complain. On any given night, one of them will refuse to eat.

Take pasta night. Eighteen-month-old Ned is the hardest to please. He eyes every food suspiciously. When he spots something he doesn't want, he'll scream, "No, no, no." Now and then, he simply says "Yuck" and drops food on the floor.

The two older kids are not much better. Three-year-old Drew doesn't like smooth rigatoni; he likes it with ridges. Naturally, his older sister, Beth, age four, wants smooth rigatoni. Even though Katy wants them to eat, she refuses to cook two different kinds of pasta.

To sidestep the pasta battle, Katy searched for the magical pasta shape both kids would eat. She tried everything from farfalle to ziti, without success. With each taste test, whenever Drew liked something, Beth didn't.

"It's enough to make you crazy," says Katy.

Instead of giving up, one day Katy and Ralph tried a new strategy. Drew and Beth would take turns choosing pasta. At first, neither child was thrilled, but soon it quelled their endless complaints. Katy and Ralph relish the truce (although they expect that one day soon Ned will start eating pasta too and upset the compromise). Still, they are perplexed. They describe themselves as "eating almost everything." Katy says, sighing in bewilderment, "We know it's not genetic. How did we end up with three picky eaters?"

Ralph and Katy are not alone. There are roughly nine million picky eaters under the age of five living in the United States today, and each one is picky in his or her own way.

While fussy eating is both common and normal in young children, some take it to amazing extremes, eating only a few select foods. More typical are kids who reject homemade chicken nuggets but eat store-bought, those who eat fruits but not vegetables, those who drink milk but refuse solid foods, or those who drink juice and refuse milk. The variations of what kids eat or don't eat are endless.

Day after day, some picky eaters eat little or nothing, while others eat well but only if offered one of a small number of foods they like. Whatever the pattern of saying no to food, the parents' struggle to help their children eat better is always the same.

Regardless of whether picky eating is a minor daily irritant or a potential threat to a child's health, it's natural for parents to worry. Most suspect there must be something they can do to make life easier for themselves and their picky eaters. Knowing exactly what that is, though, can be tricky. There are lots of pieces to the puzzle of understanding why a child refuses food. A maze of influences—developmental, biological, and environmental—affect a child's appetite and food choices.

Influences

Kids are different from one another and from one age to the next. Max refuses meat and chicken, loves salad and bread, and can't get enough cucumbers. Josh eats only pale-colored foods: cheese, yogurt, peeled apples, potatoes, and chicken. Amanda constantly drinks milk and juice but barely eats anything.

Can parents make sense out of their children's eating? In my work, the first step to finding solutions is to help parents recognize what is special and different about their child. To find the answer, I consider the influences of developmental stage, life experience, biology, and personality. Each one can support or interfere with healthy, hearty eating.

DEVELOPMENT

A child experiences mealtimes differently depending on his age and stage of development. For example, two-year-old Sam's parents were surprised and worried when his eating pattern changed. They said, "Things aren't the same. Sam was fun to feed when he was a baby. Back then, he ate *everything*. Now he barely eats anything." Although difficult to live with, mealtime tantrums are normal behavior for contrary two-year-olds.

During the second year of life the growth rate slows down and awkward attempts at independence begin. Not only do toddlers eat erratically when they do eat, but they want to do it *their* way.

The classic advice to ignore your child's food refusals applies to toddlers. Many parents justifiably find this impossible. Toddlers can be tough to ignore. The key to making the advice work depends on learning how to *act* like you don't care. Chapter 5,

"Fussy Toddlers and Preschoolers," describes the details about how toddlers demand attention and how best to respond.

For most toddlers, picky eating is an obnoxious but normal stage. Two simple rules apply: give toddlers choices and set limits.

PARENTS BEWARE
Toddlers have multiple ways of saying no to food

The "no" stage lasts about a year and moves through three stages:

- **Nonsense "no"** is playful and experimental. It doesn't necessarily express dislike or resistance. It's more about seeing what happens with a response of "no."
- **Defiant "no"** is a test of limits and power. Giving a child appropriate choices empowers her to express appropriate preferences and avoids potential showdowns.
- **Reasonable "no"** is less common, less intense, and does express personal preferences. At this stage, it's good to dig deeper. Talk to a child and find out *why* she said no.

With babies, handling picky eating is less straightforward. When food refusals start at an early age, immature eating skills are often to blame. In order to eat, babies first need to learn how. Some do it easily and happily while others resist and struggle. Young children vary a great deal in their readiness for solid foods.

Babies born early and those with medical complications are at risk for immature development. They often don't follow the typical schedule for such learning skills as walking, talking, and eating. Regardless of the cause, a child with a lag in eating or self-feeding skills is more likely to reject food.

Parents who realize there's a lag in a child's eating skills may be tempted to push harder to help their child catch up. Oddly enough, this often makes things worse. If a baby resists eating food from a spoon, holding down his arms in order to pry in extra spoonfuls isn't the solution. If a baby gags when eating stage three baby foods, giving these and other difficult foods won't help. In fact, it is likely to increase the gagging and may possibly lead to vomiting. When a child has immature eating skills, a gentle approach works best.

Meals are happier and more productive when parents are able to recognize typical behaviors for their child's development stage and adjust the pace of feeding to match the child's comfort level. Sometimes this means advancing food textures through smaller steps instead of big leaps. Even though timing varies, children eventually learn how to eat. In the meantime, keeping early eating experiences positive avoids negative associations with food. Chapter 3, "Feeding Skills," and chapter 8, "Food Textures and Flavors" offer suggestions.

Handling food refusals in children with developmental delays, aversions, or other special needs is also less straightforward. Parents may find that:

- it's harder to distinguish the difference between a child who needs help and one who is testing limits.
- picky eating patterns are more extreme. Instead of changeable and time-limited food jags, food preferences are narrow, fixed, and longer-lasting.

Autistic children often adopt rigid food routines, eating the same ten foods day in and day out. Chapter 12, "Feeding a Child with Special Needs," describes some of the strategies used to overcome slow food progressions or rigid food preferences.

BIOLOGY

From a medical perspective, poor growth, not poor appetite, is the classic sign that a child needs help. Although poor appetite and poor growth usually go together, there are exceptions.

Three-year-old Adam amazed everyone with his giant-size appetite, eating twice as much as other kids his age. Still, he remained the smallest in his group. The mountains of food Adam devoured did not help him. Adam's problem was digestion, the leading biological cause of poor growth in children.

The classic signs of a digestive problem are diarrhea or vomiting. It turned out that Adam had celiac disease, which caused him to have diarrhea whenever he ate food that contained the protein in wheat—gluten. That meant it was necessary to avoid a long list of common foods, including pasta, bread, and most crackers and cereals. Once he eliminated all foods that contained gluten, Adam's diarrhea stopped and he began to gain weight.

Of course, a serious condition is not always to blame. Because babies and young children have immature digestive systems, they are very susceptible to digestive problems—short bouts of diarrhea and vomiting are common. Fortunately, because of the short duration of these bouts, they rarely have a lasting effect on a child's growth or appetite.

It's long-term conditions that are more problematic. Any ongoing condition that causes a child to associate pain or discomfort with eating can eventually lead to food refusals. This can happen with mild digestive problems, such as reflux, constipation, or, in some cases, allergies, as well as with mechanical problems involving eating or swallowing. These are discussed in chapter 11, "Food Allergies and Digestion Problems."

Children with serious growth or feeding problems often have an underlying medical condition. Researchers report that a high percentage of children seen in medical specialty clinics such as pulmonary and GI (gastroenterology) have feeding problems. This is not surprising. Any number of medical conditions increase a young child's risk for problems with feeding or growth. Obvious problems such as cleft lip or cleft palate make eating more difficult. Less obvious are conditions that increase a child's calorie needs. These include prematurity, cerebral palsy, cystic fibrosis, and some congenital heart problems.

Because the number of children with feeding problems and medical risks has increased in recent years, more services are available. Human biology is complex. Understanding how much of a child's growth or feeding problem is inherent rather than acquired is always a challenge, but more so when a child has a medical condition.

BEYOND DIGESTION

Physiological conditions that can affect a child's eating are

- Prematurity
- Allergies
- Cerebral palsy
- Chronic infections
- Cystic fibrosis
- Congenital heart disease

See chapter 12, "Feeding a Child with Special Needs," for details.

PERSONALITY AND LIFE EXPERIENCE

In one study, parents of picky eaters cited personality traits that are common among difficult-to-feed children. Again and again, different parents used the same words: "stubborn," "moody," "socially intense," and "easily distracted."

Such common personality traits among difficult-to-feed children suggest that some are born to be fussy eaters. Of course, this knowledge doesn't help parents deal with day-to-day issues. In this study, learning techniques for handling food refusals eased the problem. (For examples of these techniques, read chapter 10, "Mealtime Do's and Don'ts." There's no doubt that biology influences a child's personality. From an academic perspective, the problem is pinpointing where this influence begins and ends.

Generally, researchers point to how life experiences affect eating. These experiences begin at birth. Miraculous, life-saving experiences for newborns and young children are more common than ever. But there is a downside. Medical interventions around the mouth (ventilators, tracheotomies, or nasogastric tubes) can cause discomfort that leads to kids rejecting food or anything that comes into or near the mouth. Professionals call this avoidance behavior. To help children overcome food refusals, therapists often use techniques based on theories of sensory integration dysfunction. For more information on how sensory integration affects eating, see chapter 8, "Food Textures and Flavors."

Family, Friends, and Peers

Defying a long-standing family tradition, five-year-old Song Woo turns up her nose at rice every day. Despite generations of rice-eating ancestors and years of bribes and threats, Song's refusal to eat rice is still going strong. She prefers pizza and spaghetti.

Song's family can't understand why she refuses rice when everyone else in her house eats it daily. Her grandmother won't give up. She uses various tactics to entice Song. Most of the time, her grandmother employs a simple bribe: "If you eat your rice, I will buy you a toy."

Song Woo's grandmother is not alone. Countless caregivers use games, tricks, and bribes to help a child eat, and in the short term they often work. But those well-intentioned bribes and cute games have unintentional consequences: over time, these kids tend to turn away from the food again. Song Woo's grandmother may convince her granddaughter to eat rice in order to get a new toy, but in the long run it increases the odds that Song will like toys and dislike rice.

For young children, eating is never solely about food or nourishment. Meals are a setting for social and physical development. Children learn whether eating is pleasant or unpleasant, which foods to like or dislike, and the consequences of eating or not eating. Sometimes adults teach these lessons without knowing it.

- If a father consistently ignores his baby's signals for "no more" and persists in prying extra spoonfuls of peas through his pursed lips, the baby learns that eating is no fun. He associates tension and discomfort with eating peas, and possibly eating in general.
- If a toddler refuses waffles and his mom offers cereal, or if when he refuses peas his mom offers carrots, a pattern emerges. Soon a toddler learns that if he refuses one food he will get another.
- A preschooler realizes that if she doesn't finish her pancakes, her mother becomes upset. This makes it harder for her to recognize whether she should eat the pancakes because she is hungry or to please her mother.

Even before they begin to talk, young children learn by watching and listening, and are amazingly aware of the social rules and expectations surrounding food. Most two-years-olds recognize cake as a party food and know that desserts are eaten after vegetables. They know which foods are popular in the family and learn the consequences of eating or refusing foods.

Because children learn about food by mimicking others, role models are important. Young children often act as mirrors, reflecting back what they see or don't see. When parents want to make meals better, watching what a child reflects back is a good place to begin.

One mother, Lisa, came to see me when her fourteen-month-old son, Gregory, was not attempting to feed himself like other children his age. From talking to her friends, she knew that other children Gregory's age behaved differently at meals; they were at least trying to eat by themselves. Gregory's play skills were typical for his age, suggesting he had the motor skills he needed to feed himself. Yet when Lisa described Gregory's meals, it seemed that Gregory rarely watched anyone else eat.

Lisa was trying to lose weight. Even though she fed her son regular meals, throughout the day she didn't eat. She saved her calories for an evening meal with her husband. Lisa had assumed that the only important thing was to feed her son healthy foods. It had never occurred to her that Gregory needed to watch *her* eat.

When she realized her own eating style might be influencing her son, she decided to be more social. She began eating with Gregory and joined a playgroup that included lunch with other children and adults. A few weeks later, after another child took a cracker off his plate, Gregory began trying to feed himself.

Role models also motivate kids to try new foods. Watching someone savor each bite of a cookie, sandwich, or fruit helps create a desire for that food. Studies show that a young child's food rejection drops when others are eating the same food. As children grow older, siblings and peers are more powerful models than adults are. Children often accept a food if they see a peer or older sibling eating it.

By the time they are preschoolers, kids are generally more open to new foods and following other kids' leads. In one study, four-year-old day-care children were grouped at tables according to their favorite vegetable. A child whose favorite vegetable was broccoli was seated at a table where everyone's favorite vegetable was carrot. Within two weeks carrots replaced broccoli as the child's favorite vegetable. In another study, preschool children watched cartoons with characters eating unfamiliar vegetables: kale, Swiss chard, and kohlrabi. Each classroom watched a cartoon with characters eating only one of the vegetables. Later, in the cafeteria, when the children were offered all three vegetables, they selected the vegetable they had seen in their classroom cartoon.

Watching others also teaches children what not to eat. Comments, facial expressions, and body language send messages. Unaware, a mother who hates spinach may dutifully feed it to her child, but with a facial grimace. It is no surprise when the child, like her mother, hates spinach.

While young children develop picky eating habits on their own, the interactions between a child and family can magnify the problem. Exploring the social dimensions around eating is one way to help picky eaters become less picky. Be practical in considering social interactions: *family* means all peers, siblings, or adults who regularly eat with or feed a young child. Anyone actively involved with the child's eating counts!

Food, Anywhere, Anytime

Picky eating is about more than individual children or their families. It's also a phenomenon—a sign of the times. The reality is that it is easy to constantly say no to food and survive.

Today, the United States offers a wonderland of food choices, unimaginable to earlier generations or to those from less fortunate parts of the world. There is a story about a Russian immigrant who, having lived through food lines and shortages, fainted from shock the first time she stepped into an American supermarket.

In the 1980s supermarkets had roughly ten thousand items on their shelves. Now the number has zoomed upward to fifty thousand. Does anyone have the time or energy to look at fifty thousand items when they go grocery shopping? Given the availability of so much food, it's easy to imagine time-squeezed adults or sensitive children being overwhelmed by the sheer volume of choices.

The explosion of food options doesn't stop at the supermarket. Most of us can find food at almost any time and any place. These days, food that used to take an hour to prepare can be hot and ready to eat after seconds in the microwave. Years ago, knowing how to cook and prepare food was essential. Today it is optional. We can always get hot food by picking up the phone, ordering online, stopping at a fast-food restaurant drive-through window, or zapping a frozen dinner in the microwave.

And since getting food whenever we want it is easier than ever, fewer families regularly sit down together for a meal. Even for those that do, snacks are available throughout the day. The calories children take in through snacks rather than meals has climbed steadily over the last twenty years.

The overabundance of food, along with a shortage of time, has not only changed *what* children eat but also *how, where,* and *when.* Increasingly we eat while doing something unrelated to food. We watch TV and eat, or drive and eat, or read our e-mail and eat.

In our fast-paced world, doing two things at once seems like a great timesaver. But there is a price. Our attention has become less focused on mealtimes, and we disconnect, at least in part, to the sensations of eating. We ignore the taste, texture, and feeling of foods going through our body, and are inattentive to the internal signals that we have eaten too much or too little. This leads to trouble.

Studies of people with eating disorders show that their eating is often unrelated to internal body signals. Their desire to eat is not triggered by hunger but rather by external cues such as seeing real food or an image of food or being bored or upset. In contrast, people with normal weight regulation are more likely to eat based on internal body signals.

Researchers have found that children improve their ability to self-regulate calories (that is, not eating more or less than is healthy) when they are encouraged to recognize signs of hunger or fullness. Interestingly, according to one study young children were better at self-regulating calories than the adults were.

For picky eaters, the *how* of feeding is key. The parents I see focus on the *what*. They worry about nutrition, the lack of protein, complex carbohydrates, vitamins, and minerals in their child's food choices. I urge them to step back and look at the big picture. There is no denying the importance of good nutrition for health, but equally important are the conditions under which children eat. Letting your children eat while watching television may not seem so terrible. Yet study after study links an increase in the number of hours spent watching television with a greater risk for eating problems. For young children, television is a distraction; it leads to a mind-body disconnection with the physical sensations of eating.

Social scientists describe food preferences as a *learned behavior*. How can we learn to eat well when we don't focus on what we are doing?

There are connections between picky eating and eating disorders. For both, incidence is lower when food choices are limited.

The blessings of abundance come with a price. Affluent countries have greater numbers of people with eating disorders. Choice brings complexity.

According to researchers, we can help our picky children eat more wholesome foods by limiting choices, reducing distractions, and offering food at regular times. To help children avoid eating too much or too little, we need to encourage them to recognize sensations of hunger and satiety and trust that they can do it. In a world where too much bad food is available at any time and any place, this is a big challenge.

Picky Eating—A Major or Minor Problem?

Does a child with a picky appetite have an eating disorder? Probably not. Finicky eating is part of normal development for young children, especially toddlers. Researchers estimate that more than 45 percent of young children are fussy eaters. For this reason, parents who complain to their pediatricians often get no support for their worries.

Feeding disorders exist in young children, but there's a tendency to avoid using labels such as anorexia or failure-to-thrive unless a child needs hospitalization. Young children vary in their eating skills and behaviors and have the potential to outgrow their problems. In their book *Childhood Feeding Disorders,* Jurgen Kedesdy and Karen Budd write: "It should be emphasized that no single item or set of items identifies a child as having a feeding disorder." As a result, referrals for a medical evaluation have traditionally been made for children whose poor eating causes a problem with growth.

Yet an increasing number of children have problems with feeding that may not be serious enough to warrant hospitalization, but are difficult for parents to handle without help. A growing number of programs offer parents services aimed at helping them confront day-to-day food refusals, and children who act out during meals, vomit regularly, or have difficulty with chewing, swallowing, or self-feeding.

The following list of questions reflects the broader range of problems that parents face and that feeding specialists address. If you have concerns about your child's eating, answer the following questions as a first step. This will help you pinpoint problem areas.

IS PICKY EATING A PROBLEM?

When you answer the questions below, keep in mind that they are a general guide and not a means to diagnose feeding problems. In the last chapter of this book, you will find "The PEACH Survey." This questionnaire was specifically designed to help parents decide whether to see a team of feeding specialists. (You'll learn more about what a feeding team does in that same chapter.)

STARTING POINT
- When did your child's problems with eating start? Did they start before the age of nine months?

GROWTH
- *Is your child underweight? To be more precise, is his/her weight for height below the fifth percentile on standard growth charts?
- *Has your child's rate of growth dropped dramatically for no obvious reason? The most common reason is an illness. (Children typically recover weight loss associated with illness quickly.)

> ## HEALTHY WEIGHT?
>
> Does your child have a healthy weight? Gain a better understanding of your child's growth pattern. See chapter 2, "Understanding Growth," for details.

Sensory or Motor Development
- *Does your child have problems with chewing or swallowing?
- *Is your child not eating table foods by the first birthday?
- Is your child not drinking from a cup by sixteen months?
- *Does your child regularly gag or vomit when eating?
- Are your child's self-feeding skills less advanced than those of other children of the same age?
- Does your child reject a specific group of foods (all having the same texture, flavor, or temperature)?
- *Does your child "fall apart" and throw tantrums when offered new foods?

> ## SENSITIVE KIDS
>
> When kids are overly sensitive to the physical properties of food, or have difficulty handling food, eating is less enjoyable. Read more about the sensory and motor connections to eating in chapter 3, "Feeding Skills," and chapter 8, "Food Textures and Flavors."

Social Interactions
- Do meals drag on, lasting longer than thirty minutes?
- Do other family members and caregivers describe your child as difficult to feed?
- Does your child act out during meals (have tantrums or throw food or dishes)?
- Does your family argue about food or feeding?

- Does your child refuse to self-feed even though he/she is able to do it?
- Does your child pouch food in the mouth and not swallow?
- *Does your child eat fewer than three times a day?

SIGNS OF TROUBLE

When kids act out with food, or meals drag on and on, something needs to change. For ideas on how to get things back on track, read chapter 9, "Family Influences," and chapter 10, "Mealtime Do's and Don'ts."

If you answered yes to two or more questions or *any* of the questions preceded with an asterisk (*), your child's fussy eating may be more than a passing stage. The information in this book won't replace the benefits from seeking individualized care. However, it will increase your awareness of the techniques and therapies used to help children overcome eating problems.

Regardless of the severity of your child's pickiness, before you can help your child to eat better, you may need to know more about how children learn to eat and the stumbling blocks they sometimes encounter. Because good growth is an integral part of good health, understanding how growth patterns affect appetite is the logical place to begin. As you read through the maze of influences that might lead your child to say no to food, you'll gain perspective and insights on how to better handle your child's picky eating.

Understanding Growth

Weight and height measurements taken during a child's physical do more than signal a need for bigger car seats. Throughout childhood, physicians use growth as a health indicator. It confirms that important changes are taking place inside the body: billions of cells are multiplying, neurons are firing, and organs are maturing—on schedule and as expected.

Growth is inextricably linked to a child's overall development. As a result, when parents complain that a child is not eating well, most doctors and dietitians first look at growth rather than appetite to answer the question of whether a picky eater is eating enough. From a medical perspective, it's poor growth rather than poor appetite that is a cause for concern.

Before handling your child's pickiness or other eating problems, it's important to determine how well your child is growing.

Fluctuations

Children don't simply grow bigger. They change in shape as well as size, with different parts of the body sometimes growing faster and sometimes slower, depending on age. As the pace and pattern of growth change, eating patterns fluctuate, causing some parents to suspect a problem when none exists. Countless children with seemingly poor appetites and shifting body proportions are quite healthy.

As a baby, six-month-old Jason had the typical proportions: a big head, a plump middle, and short, stumpy legs. Back then, his mother enjoyed pinching his meaty thighs and imagined that someday he would grow up to be stocky and solid, just like his dad.

A year later, Jason was a more finicky eater and his mother was disappointed that his thighs looked noticeably leaner. She worried that this was evidence that he was not getting the nutrition he needed.

But there was no need to worry. The changes in Jason's body were normal. After the first year of life, and just in time to start walking, the proportions of the arms and legs to the trunk change. The long bones in the arms and legs begin to grow faster. This proportional shape shifting makes toddlers and preschoolers look longer and leaner than babies.

Researchers and artists have studied the changes in body proportions throughout life. The chart on page 22 illustrates how body proportions change with age.

Along with shifts in body proportions come changes in the rate of growth. Even though children grow constantly, they don't do so at an even, steady pace. Normally the growth rate drops dramatically after the first year of life and does not speed up again until puberty. This is true for both weight and height.

The fastest growth coincides with the ages when children's appetites are at their best. Surveys find that among parents of babies, 80 percent report that their babies have good appetites while only 20 percent of parents with preschoolers have such rosy

FIGURE 1

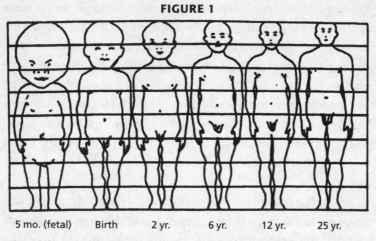

| 5 mo. (fetal) | Birth | 2 yr. | 6 yr. | 12 yr. | 25 yr. |

Adapted from *The Development and Growth of the External Dimensions of the Human Body in the Fetal Period* by Scammon, R.E., and L.A. Calkins. Copyright © 1929 by the University of Minnesota. Used with permission.

reports about their children's appetites. Along with the natural drop in growth rate typically comes a drop in appetite, alarming parents, often unnecessarily.

HOW KIDS GROW

Two-month-old babies grow at lightning speed, outgrowing clothes in a matter of months. Normally babies double their body size within the first four to six months of life. Afterward, their growth continues at a slightly slower pace until the first birthday. From then on the growth rate drops further.

Data collected on thousands of children over the last century illustrates how dramatic this drop in growth rate is. An average two-month-old gains six ounces in a week. By age three, a child takes four times longer to gain six ounces. Instead of a week, it takes a month. The chart on page 23 compares typical weight gains for children at different ages.

WEEKLY WEIGHT GAINS

Typical weight gains for the average-size child (growing at the fiftieth percentile on the growth charts developed by the National Center for Health Statistics)

Age (months)	Weight (ounces)
1–6	5–6
6–12	3–5
12–15	2
15–36	1.5
36–48	1.2

NOTE: Children who are above or below the fiftieth percentile will have different weight gains at each age but will follow the same pattern.

The slowdown in growth affects height as well as weight. In the first year of life a baby may grow ten inches, then, in the second year, only four inches. By the third and fourth years, the gains in height slow down to just less than three inches each year.

✕ *If you are worried about your child's growth, talk to your pediatrician. After the first birthday, pediatricians often weigh and measure children every six months up to age two, and once a year after that.*

Understanding Growth Charts

If you keep a log of your child's weight and height measurements you can see just how much your child grows from year to year. But if you plot those same measurements on a standard growth chart, you'll learn much more. Growth charts are a useful screening tool that answers such basic questions as:

- How fast or slow is my child's weight or height growing compared to other children his or her age and gender?
- Is my child taller or shorter than other boys or girls his age?
- Is my child thinner or fatter?

If a child's growth rate is average, the measurements plot parallel to the percentile lines. When the plotted line drops down from the percentile lines a child's growth rate is slower than average (see fig. 2), and when it rises above the percentile line the growth rate is faster (see fig. 3). This pattern is often seen in babies born prematurely who go through a period of rapid growth, which helps them to "catch up" to other children their age who were not premature.

To compare a child's weight or height to other children of the same age, find the closest percentile line (look for the dark, heavy lines). When a child's weight for his age is at the sixtieth percentile on the growth chart, it means that compared to one hundred other boys his age, forty would weigh more and sixty would weigh less.

Since pediatricians normally track a child's growth as part of routine care, you don't need to on your own unless you'd like to keep a close watch.

WHAT'S NORMAL AND WHAT'S NOT

Children who stand out as being noticeably smaller or taller than their peers attract attention and concern. Yet such comparisons, which are based on a child's weight or height for age, often reflect family genes rather than health problems.

Healthy children come in a variety of sizes. Four-year-olds can vary by as much as fifteen pounds in weight and six inches in height without appearing to be abnormally tall, heavy, or thin—as long as their weight is in proportion to their height.

FIGURE 2

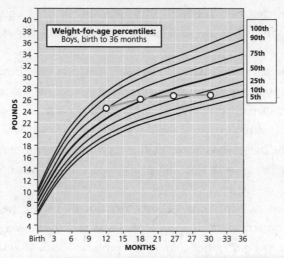

Adapted from the National Centers for Disease Control growth charts, published May 30, 2000. Available online at www.cdc.gov.

FIGURE 3

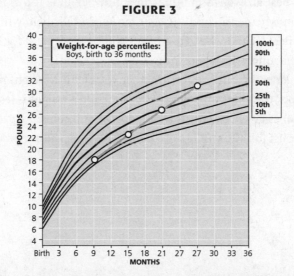

Adapted from the National Centers for Disease Control growth charts, published May 30, 2000. Available online at www.cdc.gov.

When Amanda looked over the class of preschoolers, she realized that her daughter, Kim, was the smallest child in the room. Until then she had never worried about her daughter's size.

Minutes after leaving the school, Amanda called the doctor. He assured her that Kim's growth was fine. It was true that Kim was small compared to other girls her age. She was at the fifth percentile for both weight and height. But it was nothing new; she had always been small. Everything else was normal, including her growth rate and proportions. There was no need to worry.

To check Kim's proportions, her doctor used a weight-for-length growth chart. It specifically looks at a child's weight in relation to *height* rather than *age*. Compare Kim's growth charts. The first compares her weight to that of other girls her age (see fig. 4). The second compares her weight to her height (see fig. 5).

The best answer to the question "how small is too small?" is based on whether a child's *weight for height* falls below the fifth percentile. (A child who is too heavy will have a weight for height above the ninety-fifth percentile.)

For general guidelines on whether your child's weight may be low, check the chart on page 28. If your child's weight is less than the number given, discuss it with a doctor and consult a pediatric nutritionist for ideas on how to boost his or her calorie intake.

FIGURE 4

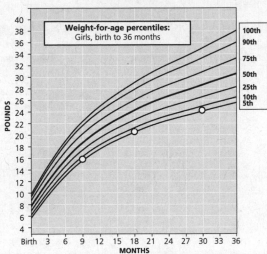

Adapted from the National Centers for Disease Control growth charts, published May 30, 2000. Available online at www.cdc.gov.

FIGURE 5

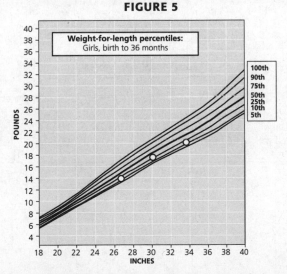

Adapted from the National Centers for Disease Control growth charts, published May 30, 2000. Available online at www.cdc.gov.

WORRISOME WEIGHTS

Based on weights for lengths/heights falling below the fifth percentile.

Length/Height (inches)	Girls Weight (pounds)	Boys Weight (pounds)
30	19.8	20.2
31	20.8	21.3
32	22	22.5
33	23.25	23.5
34	24.3	24.5
35	25.4	25.75
36	26.5	27
37	27.5	28.2
38	29	29.5
39	30.3	30.8
40	31	31.8
41	31.5	32
42	33.75	34.5
43	35	36
44	36.75	37.8
45	38.5	39.8
46	40.25	41.2
47	42.5	43
48	44	44.5

NOTE: Length is measured with a child lying down. Height (stature) is measured with a child standing.

BODY MASS INDEX (BMI)

Another measure for assessing whether a child is too heavy or too thin involves using the Body Mass Index (BMI). The BMI is used differently with children than it is with adults. Children are still growing and the percentage of body fat changes as they mature. Because body fatness is part of the BMI calculation, the numbers that define healthy weight for children change according to age and gender. Compare how the numbers change for two-year-old and four-year-old boys.

For a two-year-old boy: Overweight means having a BMI of 19.3 or more. Underweight means having a BMI of 14.7 or less.

For a four-year-old boy: Overweight means having a BMI of 17.8 or more. Underweight means having a BMI of 14 or less.

Information on how to use the BMI in children is available online. You'll find it at www.cdc.gov.

Some parents rejoice when their child gains an ounce of weight or grows half an inch. But regardless of whether there's a concern about a child's growth, it pays to look further than the latest weight or height.

From time to time, it's good to review a series of measurements. Multiple measurements paint a picture of a child's growth over time and help answer a broader question: Is a child's growth too fast, too slow, or just right?

A common definition of a growth pattern that is just right is one that follows the curve on the chart. This is true even when a child is bigger or smaller than other children of the same age. A small child whose growth is stable and follows the normal curve is considered to be healthy.

Likewise, there are healthy children whose growth pattern deviates from the standard. Big babies don't always grow into big toddlers. It's not unusual to see shifts in a child's growth pattern, especially during the first two years of life. These shifts stand out when one looks carefully at the dark, heavy lines on growth charts that mark major percentiles (such as the tenth, twenty-fifth, fiftieth, seventy-fifth, and ninetieth) and indicate a child's size relative to other kids the same age. Yet such drop-offs should not be automatically dismissed.

A child's growth may slow down temporarily because of illness or poor appetite. Or it may be due to something more fundamental. Genes and chromosomes exert a powerful influence on a child's growth.

Any prolonged downward shift in a child's growth pattern should be discussed with a doctor. At times, too steep a drop in growth rate reflects a condition that requires medical intervention.

As a baby, Jose was so big that his parents nicknamed him Gordo (which means "fat" in Spanish). Two years later, the nickname no longer applied. Jose's growth had fallen steadily, crossing two channels on the growth chart. It turned out that Jose's tonsils were swollen, which made swallowing painful. He needed surgery to have his tonsils and adenoids removed. After the surgery, Jose was able to swallow more comfortably and his growth rate resumed a normal curve.

While it is easy to compare a child's size in relation to other children, it is harder to recognize when a child's growth rate changes. The best way to notice these changes is by tracking a child's growth over time.

Complications in Using Growth Charts

Growth charts are a screening tool and not a standard to which every child must conform. There are instances when a healthy child's growth doesn't match the typical pattern on the chart.

When a child's growth doesn't match the chart, consider the following:

- **Family Patterns**

  The height of parents is an obvious indicator of a child's growth potential. But there are other family growth patterns that may be important. Constitutional Growth Delay (CGD) is often hereditary and causes children to be "late bloomers." Although they often attain normal height as adults, growth is slower during early childhood. Catch-up growth occurs after puberty, which is later than usual.

- **Health**

  Any condition that affects a child's health can affect appetite or growth. Asthma and eczema can simply reduce a child's appetite, while heart or lung conditions can increase calorie needs. Children with neurological problems as well as recognized syndromes often have poor growth. Turner, Noonan, Down, and Russell-Silver syndromes all impact growth. See chapter 12, "Feeding a Child with Special Needs," for more information.

- **Appearance**

  A child's weight reflects a shifting body composition of fluids, fat, muscle mass, and skeleton. Whenever a child's body composition differs from the norm, growth charts can be misleading. Muscle weighs more than fat. As a result, an athletic child with more muscle mass and less fat than average looks overweight on the growth chart. For such a child, physical appearance contradicts the chart. The child looks solid and muscular rather than overweight.

Despite some limitations, growth charts remain a valuable tool for monitoring a child's health.

Predicting the Future

Americans have been growing taller. Over the last century, generation after generation has grown taller than their parents. But researchers believe this trend is over. Today, Junior growing taller than Dad is not as likely as it was fifty years ago.

Better living conditions help children grow taller than their parents. During the past century, rising standards of living in the United States brought better health to millions, and with it came big gains in both life expectancy and linear growth. A series of lifestyle changes swept through the land of opportunity, helping young Americans grow taller and achieve their genetic potential. But this trend has a limit.

Researchers report that the American population has achieved the genetic potential for height. The current prediction is that as a group, future generations of Americans may grow heavier but not taller.

Parents who want to predict the adult height of their children can try one of the following formulas, with the caveat that none is guaranteed to be accurate:

- Double a boy's height at twenty-four months. Double a girl's height at eighteen months.

- Add heights of both parents, then divide by 2. If the child is a boy, add 2½ inches. If the child is a girl, subtract 2½ inches.
- For boys, adult height = 1.27 × height at 3 years + 22 inches. For girls, adult height = 1.29 × height at 3 years + 17 inches.

If you prefer someone else to do the math, try the online "Kid's Height Predictor" on WebMD.com.

Finally, once you understand your child's growth pattern, you'll be in a better position to judge the impact of your child's picky eating on his health. Adequate growth has been described as the most important developmental task of childhood. Even if your picky eater refuses vegetables, milk, or meat, as long as growth is on track, you know that he is taking in enough calories to meet his basic needs. This is important.

Do
- Expect some fluctuations in your child's appetite and growth.
- Discuss your child's growth with the pediatrician.
- Expect your child's growth pattern to be influenced by family history.
- Consider health issues that are likely to affect your child's growth.

Don't
- Be surprised if a big baby doesn't grow into a big preschooler.
- Push your child to eat more when growth is normal.
- Assume that bigger is better. A small child who is growing at a normal rate is healthy.
- Dismiss a drop-off in your child's growth without discussing it with the pediatrician.

Feeding Skills

Millions of babies progress from eating baby foods to table foods without interruption. For many parents it seems as though one day their baby is eating pureed mush, and not long after she is chomping through dry cereal and crackers.

But the truth is that the process is not simple. And when babies don't progress from one food to the next, it is impossible to help them without understanding the skills required to bite, chew, and swallow. After one begins to learn all the minute steps in this process, it seems more understandable that some children need help along the way.

This chapter examines the skills that young children need to master before they are able to eat table foods. It also looks at ideal periods for the transition from bottles to cups and the links between eating and other areas of a child's development.

Ideal Periods

For many years, experts have suggested that there are windows of opportunity when children can learn, adapt, or develop new skills easily. If they miss these "critical periods," it becomes harder or even impossible for them to pick up these skills later.

This idea is an old one. We know that when a child has a lazy eye, she needs an eye patch early; otherwise, it remains a lifelong condition. We also know that those who learn a second language after puberty generally speak with an accent.

When it comes to food habits, there is some truth to the idea of critical periods. But because children have plasticity, and a remarkable ability to adapt, the word *critical* seems too strong. "Ideal periods" is better.

There are periods in development during which a child is most open to forming new food habits. Here are the big four I see:

- **Weaning**—Transition off bottle or breast
- **Drinking Milk**—Transition to a cup
- **Sitting at the Table**—Establishing a place for eating
- **Chewing**—Learning to chew solid foods

Weaning—Transition off Bottle or Breast

✕ *Ideal Time: If growth is normal, begin around a baby's first birthday.*

Weaning off the bottle is easy before fifteen months of age but much harder ten months later. Babies are more flexible, so taking bottles away soon after the first birthday makes it easy. By age two, children are more rigid and resistant to changes that they do not initiate. Taking a bottle away from a two-year-old is noticeably harder.

Jennifer and Bill had struggled to take bottles away from two of their four children—the older boys. I suggested that they wean their younger twins earlier. They gave it a try. When their bottles were taken away at fourteen months, the twins barely fussed. Jennifer and Bill were amazed at the difference.

Drinking Milk—Transition to a Cup

✕ **Ideal Time:** *If growth is normal, offer sips of water around seven months. By eleven or twelve months, offer formula in a cup.*

Whether milk or juice comes in cups or bottles doesn't matter much to a one-year-old. But children change. Babies accustomed to drinking juice only from a cup and drinking milk only from a bottle typically refuse to drink milk from a cup as toddlers. It's better to introduce breast milk, formula, or a milklike drink (yogurt smoothie) in a cup early (before one year or soon after). Parents who do not introduce a milklike drink in the cup early on often find that they take the child's milk away when they take the bottle away.

Sitting at the Table—Establishing a Place for Eating

✕ **Ideal Time:** *When babies are able to sit up—often between six and eight months.*

Once children are able to move around independently, it becomes harder to have them sit for meals. It's best to establish the habit early. When it's time to eat, put your baby in the high chair. This creates the idea that there is a special place for eating. Babies go along with this idea, but defiant toddlers don't. If you wait too long and don't establish this habit, your child will be more likely to fuss at every meal.

Chewing—Learning to Chew Solid Foods

✕ *Ideal Time: After babies learn to move their tongues from side to side—often but not always between nine and twelve months.*

Before older babies can chew solid foods they need to move their tongues from side to side and coordinate this with up-and-down jaw movements. This typically begins around nine months of age, and with continual practice over the next six months babies refine their skills and learn to eat a wide array of table foods. For some babies this process is delayed or thrown off schedule. Common reasons for this include

- illness
- aversions
- lack of experience with more difficult foods
- immature motor development

Regardless of the reason, as an older child tries to learn to bite and chew, it becomes more important to progress textures in small incremental steps and to work through a child's resistance.

Because Jordan had life-threatening allergies, his family delayed giving him solid foods until after his first birthday. At sixteen months, Jordan refused to eat anything other than the pureed baby foods with which he was familiar. A therapist helped him to overcome his resistance to new foods and to learn how to bite and chew more difficult foods by

- strengthening his mouth muscles with nonfood activities such as blowing bubbles.
- motivating him to *want* to try new foods by offering them in

a playgroup with other children or when his older brother was present.

- making new foods easier to eat by offering them in a gradual progression that incorporated texture-to-texture and flavor-to-flavor strategies (see chapter 8, "Food Textures and Flavors").

And despite the focus on providing increasingly more difficult foods, food was *always* offered in a low-key, noncoercive manner. Six months later, Jordan was happily eating table foods.

Links Between Skills

As children grow and develop, skill differences emerge. Two-year-old Amanda uses more words and speaks more clearly than her three-year-old playmate Lois. To further complicate matters, it's also true that a problem in one area of development sometimes spills over into another. The most obvious links with feeding involve motor skills and speech.

MOVING AND EATING

A child who is slow to walk or sit is likely to need more time to learn how to eat foods that require biting and chewing. Amy and her twin sister, Anna, barely seemed like twins. Because Amy had a heart defect and digestive problems, she had been in and out of the hospital. When her mom counted up the days, it added up to two months in the hospital. At their first birthday, Amy was not only smaller than her sister, she was barely sitting up and, sadly, not able to eat her birthday cake. But, with time, Amy made progress. Although she remained smaller than Anna, at their second birthday both girls were walking, talking, and eating their cake.

FEELING AND EATING

When a baby chews on a toy, it looks primitive and messy, but it serves an important purpose. The physical sensations that register in the baby's mouth send messages to her brain, creating important pathways. Babies who never mouth toys are more likely, months later, to have problems with food textures.

To understand how children experience and react to food sensations, it helps to see a child who, for medical reasons, is not given food by mouth early on. From watching the facial expressions of one-year-old Jason as he eats food by mouth for the first time, it seems unlikely that he really tastes the food at all. He seems so overwhelmed by the experience itself. Even though Jason has all the wiring to taste food, it's obvious that he is not yet ready to focus on this subtler dimension of food. Initially all his reactions to the food are based on tolerating the sensations in his mouth. It is only later that he seems able to discriminate the flavor of one food from that of another.

Babies are born with immature nervous systems, and this affects their reactions to stimulation. Babies can be so sensitive to sound or light that it disrupts eating. This is often true for babies who are born prematurely, but it also happens with older children who are easily distracted. Young children can also be highly sensitive to touch, clothing, food, or the taste, touch, or feel of food going into the mouth.

In helping children tolerate new foods, occupational therapists often assess how a child responds to sights, sounds, touch, and smell, and their overall body balance and awareness. These assessments form the basis for helping children feel more comfortable with the physical sensations of food.

TALKING AND EATING

The mouth moves to eat and later to talk. Because the same muscles are involved, a problem with one is often linked to a problem with the other.

The trained eye of a feeding specialist looks at details of the mouth in action: suck-and-swallow coordination, strong or weak suck, lip closure around a spoon or nipple, tongue movements in eating. These and other details provide clues as to what can help a child with feeding problems.

Dylan had impressive skills for a two-year-old. He could count to thirty and recognize both simple and complex shapes: circles, squares, triangles, cylinders, and arches. His dad, an engineer, spent many hours with him, and it was not hard to imagine how they spent their time together.

Dylan was a bright, energetic, and happy child. His dad requested a consult because Dylan did not eat well. The concern was not *how much* Dylan ate, since his growth was normal, but *what* he ate. Generally Dylan did not eat foods that required chewing. Not surprisingly, he also saw a speech therapist because his language was delayed.

Dylan's tongue movements were more primitive than those of a typical two-year-old. He barely moved his tongue from side to side, and when he did, he was not able to coordinate tongue movement with chewing. By doing exercises that encouraged Dylan to move his tongue, his eating skills soon improved. In a short time, Dylan made big improvements in both talking and eating.

PLAYING AND EATING

Play connects to eating both directly and indirectly. Clumsy toddlers gain dexterity when using a spoon and fork to feed dolls or stuffed animals.

Therapists focus a child's attention on food and make it fun by understanding his learning abilities and interests. What appears to be play is actually based on educational theories and standard-ized tests that map out when children do what. A one-year-old who is afraid to try a cracker watches a therapist feed it to a puppet. Later he imitates her, and later still he puts the cracker in his mouth. A three-year-old who is learning shapes and colors talks about the shapes and colors of the food on his plate. And so a child's tolerance to new foods is slowly expanded through play.

Surprisingly, there's also an indirect connection between play and eating. For one child, play improved all areas of his life. Je-remy was a fussy, difficult twenty-month-old. In fact, he was the grumpiest child I had ever encountered. He was diagnosed with failure-to-thrive after his growth rate dropped at nine months. The pediatrician told his parents to give him extra calories. At first, they became less strict about offering only "healthy" foods. Whatever Jeremy wanted to eat was okay. Still, he didn't gain enough weight. At meals, his parents alternately tried to push and bribe him, but finally left food on the table, and Jeremy wandered back and forth for more bites, typically dragging meals out for two hours.

When I talked to his mom, I gave her standard recommenda-tions for adding extra calories and for setting limits. These in-cluded limiting meals to thirty minutes and putting food out with the attitude "Here is your food. If you want to eat it, fine, and if you don't, that's okay too."

At the same time, a developmental educator began working with Jeremy. She brought out toys that made learning fun and motivated him to follow directions. He joined a playgroup, which helped him to learn social skills such as listening and waiting for a turn.

Jeremy's parents saw how he liked puzzles and Mr. Potato

Head, and they bought him toys that helped him to "play" more constructively. As Jeremy's attention span grew, he sat still longer during play and meals.

Within three months, Jeremy changed into a happy, pleasant little boy with a normal growth rate. Adding positive activities to Jeremy's life spilled over into mealtimes. By providing this bright little boy more stimulation and structure, Jeremy's growth and life improved.

Learning to Eat: Milestones

Milestone charts help parents recognize when kids do what. The problem, of course, is that not all children follow the schedule on the charts. When children are delayed, parents tend to fear that they will forever be behind. But it's not true; kids mature at different rates.

Specialists in child development know that a milestone chart is more than a timetable. It shows sequence and links. If your child's eating skills don't match the timeline on the chart below, focus on your child's current level of eating skills and help your child move ahead toward the next stage. The timeline is not as important as the sequence.

In addition, kids with delays catch up faster when the steps for feeding are broken down into smaller segments. For example, instead of going from purees to lumpy foods, the purees may need to be thickened first. For more information on fine-tuning food textures, see chapter 8, "Food Textures and Flavors."

LEARNING TO EAT—STEP BY STEP

When Approximate age	How Mouth and body movements/skills	What Typical foods/eating behavior
Birth through 5 months	Coordinates sucking, swallowing, and breathing. Poor control of head, neck, and trunk.	Swallows liquids.
4 months through 7 months	Begins up-and-down munching movement. Opens mouth for the spoon. Closes the upper or lower lip around the spoon. Moves food to the back of the tongue to swallow. Sits with support. Good head control. Uses whole hand to grasp objects.	Swallows liquids. Gums or mouths pureed foods.
5 months through 9 months	Closes lip on spoon to remove food. Positions food between the jaws for chewing. Follows food with eyes. Begins to sit alone without support. Begins to use a pincer grasp to pick up food.	Gums and swallows crackers. Eats pureed/mashed foods. Drinks from a cup (dribbles) held by adult. Begins self-feeding with hands.
8 months through 11 months	Uses the tongue to move food from side to side in the mouth. Begins to curve lips around the rim of the cup. Begins to chew in rotary pattern. Sits alone easily. Transfers objects from hand to mouth. Swallows with mouth closed.	Bites and chews cracker. Licks food off a spoon. Eats mashed table foods. Finger-feeds small pieces of food. Begins to experiment with spoon. Drinks from a cup with less spilling.

(continued)

When Approximate age	How Mouth and body movements/skills	What Typical foods/eating behavior
10 months through 12 months	Rotary chewing. Begins to put spoon in the mouth. Begins to hold cup (enjoys turning cup upside down).	Eats chopped food and small pieces of soft, cooked table foods. Begins self-spoon-feeding.
12 months	Picks up food with a refined pincer grasp (thumb and forefinger). Picks up and drinks from a cup (expect spills).	Bites nipples, spoons, and crunchy foods. Prefers finger foods.
15 months +	Licks lower lip with tongue. Drinks independently from a cup, holding it with one or two hands. Uses spoon to self-feed (with spills).	Bites and chews almost all cooked table foods. Eats cut-up pieces of fresh fruit. Prefers meats that don't require much chewing.
18 months +	Lips close when chewing. Uses the spoon more effectively (lifts elbow and flexes wrist). Uses words to signal "all done" or "more." Sucks through a straw.	Appetite and food preferences fluctuate.
2 years +	Uses a spoon to self-feed without spilling. Starts to use fork. No pause when moving food from side to side in the mouth.	Drinks from a cup without dribbling. Eats foods with mixed textures.
3 years +	Can clean the lips with tongue. Tongue tip elevates when swallowing. Washes and dries hands with minimal or no adult help.	Chews and swallows majority of adult foods.

SAFETY FIRST

Basic Guidelines for Feeding Young Children

Because feeding-skill maturity varies in young children, follow these precautions:

- Keep a watchful eye on young children when they eat.
- Don't allow kids to eat while they are in the car, "on the run," or moving about. The best and safest place for kids to eat is sitting down at a table.
- Modify foods to match a child's eating skills. For children under three, avoid hard foods such as nuts, raw carrots, and hard candies. Cut meats (especially hot dogs), grapes, and other risky foods into smaller, easy-to-eat pieces.
- Avoid feeding a child too soon after using rub-on teething medications. These can numb the muscles in the throat and make chewing and swallowing more difficult.

Feeding Skills and Motor Development

If you look at a box of Gerber teething biscuits, you will find guidelines on when babies are ready to eat finger foods. The guidelines don't mention age. Instead they describe skills such as crawling with the tummy off the floor and pincer grasp (holding food between the thumb and first finger). This information highlights an important fact—that a child's readiness to bite and chew foods is related to motor skills.

✕ *Use physical maturity as a guide for increasing food texture. To recognize the skills a child needs in order to advance food textures, review the guidelines in the "Learning to Eat" chart (pages 43–44).*

Rather than thinking of motor skills as being on a timetable, therapists also think of them as stages that build one upon the other. Normally, large muscles supporting the trunk mature first, thus providing a stable base for the more refined movements in the face and hands. To an untrained eye, the fine points in the development and sequence of these motor skills are easy to miss.

GAGGING

At six months, Cameron did not sit up, even with support. When the doctor took a closer look, he discovered a tight muscle in Cameron's neck (torticollis). This made it uncomfortable for him to turn his head, which in turn also affected other muscles.

Following suggestions from a physical therapist, Julia, his mom, began a regular program of massage and exercises. Gradually, Cameron stopped favoring one side and moved his head in all directions. Much to Julia's relief, a few months later, Cameron could sit up all by himself. However, she was still concerned about his eating habits.

Julia knew that other kids Cameron's age were eating dry cereal, crackers, and soft fruits. When she gave these foods to Cameron, he spit them out or choked. Julia worried that Cameron had a throat problem. Instead, she discovered that the muscles that held up his head and shoulders influenced his eating skills. For Cameron, the tight muscle in his neck contributed to delays with both sitting up and eating.

✖ *Encourage good posture to make eating easier. Swallowing is easier when your head is straight and your chin is tucked down. Experience the difference the wrong position makes. Tilt your head back and swallow. You will feel tension in your neck. If you close your jaw, swallowing becomes even more uncomfortable.*

A number of medical conditions, both serious and minor, can delay a child's physical maturity. When kids are slow to walk, talk, or eat, therapists take a closer look at muscle movements, large and small, throughout the body. How effective are the movements of the small muscles in the mouth (oral-motor) or in the hands (fine motor) or the large muscles in the legs and trunk (gross motor)? Slow motor development often affects a child's eating skills.

SWALLOWING

At two, Kelly had problems with eating and talking. She went to a feeding clinic for a work-up. This included a swallowing test that showed immature movements of her tongue. When Kelly ate she did not move her tongue from side to side or lift the tip when she swallowed.

✕ *Understand the tests that diagnose oral-motor delays. Professionals sometimes use tests to look at the three phases of swallowing. The oral phase looks at movements of food inside the mouth. Once food is pushed to the back of the tongue it triggers a reflex, which closes valves to prevent food from entering the nose or windpipe. (This is called the pharyngeal stage.) With the help of gravity and muscle contractions, food travels down the esophagus and into the stomach and concludes the final step in swallowing—the esophageal phase.*

Kelly was referred to a speech therapist, who taught her to move her tongue from side to side. In their first session, she dabbed marshmallow Fluff in the corners of Kelly's mouth and encouraged her to lick it off. Kelly liked Fluff but struggled to reach it. The next time the therapist tried the Fluff, she used a mirror so that Kelly could watch herself. This worked. The therapist also had Kelly and her mom do mouth exercises and massage at home. Within a few months, Kelly learned to use her tongue to position food between her teeth. Along with this, she gagged less and slowly began to try more table foods. Initially, Kelly had pointed to the foods she wanted to eat, but now when Kelly spoke it was easier to understand her and she could use words instead of gestures to express herself.

A careful look at how a child moves the tongue, lips, and cheeks helps a speech therapist recognize immature movements that contribute to delays. As kids improve strength and coordination of mouth movements, talking and eating improve.

✕ *Encourage mature development of mouth muscles through a drinking cup. In selecting the right cup for a child, parents usually look for those that are spill-proof, easy to drink from, and easy to clean. But this type of cup also affects calorie intake and development of mouth-muscle skills. If your child has problems gaining weight, handling food textures, or speaking, take a closer look at your child's cup. For more details on this, see chapter 7, "Making Food Desirable."*

DROOLING

Ian drooled constantly. Even though he was two years old, he had difficulty drinking from a cup of any kind and still used a bottle. He was a small, friendly boy who liked to talk, but no one outside his family understood him. He saw a speech therapist who recommended taking the bottle away to encourage mature muscle movements in his mouth. Although this did help his speech, once Ian stopped drinking from the bottle, his calorie intake plummeted and soon his growth fell off the chart. He saw a pediatric dietitian for ideas on how to boost up his calories.

✕ *If a child needs to maximize calories, be cautious about making big food changes. Maximizing oral-motor (mouth muscle) skills makes it harder for kids to take in calories. In some cases, it's best to maximize oral-motor skills without using food.*

By age two, most kids have stopped drooling. While drooling is normal and gradually goes away on its own, when kids older than two drool, it's best to explore the cause. Allergies and chronic respiratory problems lead kids to breathe through the mouth. This often extends the time they drool. Less common causes are dental problems, medication, and reflux. These possibilities can be discussed with a doctor.

Otherwise, when kids without congestion drool, the cause is related to decreased sensation in the mouth, low muscle tone, or a motor delay involving the entire body or only the mouth. Simple remedies such as reminding children to close their mouths, wiping their faces, or trying the activities listed below will help. If kids continue to drool, individual therapy will address a child's specific needs. The therapy could help a child increase overall body strength in the head, neck, shoulders, and trunk. Or it could focus on muscles in the face that control jaw stability, and lip, tongue, and cheek movements.

Ian's problem with drinking from a cup stemmed from low muscle tone in his cheeks and jaw muscles. The quality of muscle movement is determined not only by strength and coordination but also by tone, which is most likely to cause problems when it's too high or low. High muscle tone results in tight or rigid movement while low tone results in loose or floppy movement. The low tone in Ian's cheeks and mouth caused him to keep his mouth open.

SELF-FEEDING

Now and then, I see older children, two- and three-years-olds, who don't feed themselves. The first thing I look for are signs that a child is motivated to self-feed and how the parents support or encourage the child to self-feed.

Henry lived in a comfortable house with loving parents. Henry's mother described him as a wonderful little boy who played well, listened well, and slept well. There was only one problem: Henry was a terrible eater. He refused meat and vegetables, preferring sweets, snacks, and fluids. At two and a half, Henry could feed himself with his fingers and a spoon, drink from a cup, and use a straw. Despite his abilities, he much preferred to be fed and the food to be broken up for him. He also hated being messy.

Because Henry was small and his weight gain slow, his parents went along with feeding him. It was obvious that Henry *could* feed himself, he just preferred not to. For Henry, family dynamics, a minor sensory preference, and too many fluids added up to creating one terrible eater.

The changes that improved Henry's eating included cutting down on his milk consumption during the day, giving him a high-calorie drink at bedtime, having him use his hands to play in the sandbox and at a rice table, offering him more finger foods, and bringing him to a playgroup that had an organized snack session where all the kids ate the same foods at the same time. His parents were firmer about setting limits with him around food, and slowly Henry began to feed himself.

✂ *To motivate a reluctant self-feeder, use a favorite food. If a child who is able to self-feed resists, parents need to find ways to motivate him. Start with foods a child likes to eat.*

Encouragement strongly influences a child's motivation to feed herself, and child-development specialists advocate early self-feeding because it gives a child a sense of accomplishment, which improves self-esteem. Yet, there are young children who *do* lack the skills to self-feed.

Three-year-old Jackson, another boy who didn't feed himself, had a different story. Jackson loved to move. He could walk, climb stairs, jump, squat, and walk a few steps on a balance beam. When it came to moving his body, he was strong, sturdy, and coordinated. Yet these skills did not carry over to using his hands. He fumbled when putting pegs in a pegboard. He held a crayon awkwardly, and he stacked only four blocks in a tower. Jackson had problems using a spoon or fork and made a mess with finger foods. Normally his mother fed him, being careful to place food in the back of his mouth; otherwise it fell out.

✕ *As kids grow older, expect the link between motor skills and eating skills to change. The connection between gross-motor skills and eating is more pronounced for babies than for older children. Although good posture and alignment while eating are always important, the inability in an older child to walk does not affect the ability to eat.*

Jackson was big for his age—weighing forty pounds at age three. It was hard to imagine that eating was a problem for him. Yet he could not drink through a straw, and when he tried to drink from an open cup, liquid dribbled down his chin. Nonetheless, Jackson managed to drink quite well from a sippy cup. In fact, this was the secret to his robust body size. He drank milk constantly, up to half a gallon a day, plus two to three cups of juice.

Watching Jackson at mealtime made it clear that he lacked the skills needed to feed himself. When he used a spoon, he brought it straight up to his mouth, with the food falling off along the way. By age three, kids generally use a spoon effectively.

In order to learn how to manipulate objects with their hands, kids need to sit still. Jackson rarely sat still. In fact, his favorite activity was to climb and crash. Jackson's poor self-feeding was due, at least in part, to hyperactivity, a diagnosis confirmed by a neurologist.

Before he could feed himself, Jackson needed help. He had developmental delays and attended a special-needs preschool classroom with a teacher who understood his needs. A speech and occupational therapist gave specific suggestions that helped Jackson strengthen his jaw muscles and learn how to drink from an open cup as well as through a straw. He also learned to sit for longer periods of time, and slowly he learned to manipulate objects, including a spoon.

✕ *Look for adaptive devices to make eating easier. Jackson used a skid-proof mat to keep his bowl in place. For details on finding utensils that are easier to hold and dishes that make it easier to scoop food out, see chapter 7, "Making Food Desirable."*

A pediatric dietitian recommended cutting the milk down to twenty-four ounces a day. This increased Jackson's hunger for solid foods. One year later, Jackson had gained the skills he needed to eat by himself and had moved on to new challenges. He was working on speaking so that others would understand him, and he learned to listen to others and sit for longer periods of time.

Despite the pitfalls mentioned above, it is important to realize that all muscle movements don't need to be perfect. Normally, kids bumble through new movements gaining strength and coordination. Sometimes they compensate for weakness in one area with strength in another. Kids with minor problems often outgrow them.

Mouth Muscle Exercises

Use these activities to strengthen and stimulate mouth muscles. Do them before meals to stimulate and prepare the mouth or use them as an alternate way to help kids to gain the skills that make eating easier without hassling over food.

USE THAT MOUTH
Activities to strengthen the lips, cheeks, and tongue:

Blowing (Start with the easy ones and work up.)
- Play "puffy cheek" games.
- Blow paint through a straw.
- Fill a dishpan with water and a few drops of dish soap. Then blow bubbles through a straw or plastic tubing.
- Blow bubbles with the wand that comes in the bottle, then move on to bigger wands or bubble toys that require more forceful blowing.
- Blow cotton balls or feathers across a tabletop.
- Blow a tissue up into the air.
- Make sounds with whistles, noisemakers, pinwheels, or musical toys like a kazoo or a harmonica.
- Look for toys that encourage blowing or inhaling. If you find one that requires more effort than a child has, wait and try it again later.

Sucking (Experiment with tart or sour flavors.)
- Popsicles
- Drink through a straw (look for different types: long/short, thin/wide, smooth/ridges, and straight/squiggly).
- Drink from a sippy cup (spill-proof styles require a stronger suck).

- Drink from a sports bottle or novelty-shaped container such as a toy canteen.

Licking

- Sauce on a large wooden spoon
- Dab food outside your child's mouth and encourage licking the lips to get it off.
- Make silly faces in the mirror and teach your child to mimic tongue movements (in/out and side to side).

Make sounds that bring the lips together, such as *ba-ba, bo-bo, ma-ma,* and *pa-pa.*

Play games that use the lips: kisses, lip smacking, humming, and blowing raspberries.

Need more ideas? Read the book *Mouth Madness: Oral-Motor Activities for Children* by Catherine Orr, Therapy Skill Builders.

TOYS AND DEVICES THAT STIMULATE THE MOUTH

Therapists use toys and devices to help stimulate the mouth. These also make it easier for therapy to feel like play. To maximize their effectiveness, talk to a therapist for suggestions on how to best use the following for your child:

Infa-Dent Finger Toothbrush This is a soft plastic massager that fits over an adult finger. The tip has soft bristles that can be used as a toothbrush to clean teeth or massage gums. It's also used to "wake up" the mouth before feeding by stroking gums, cheeks, and tongue. Available from a pharmacy, Toys "R" Us, or

Nu-Tec Health Products, Inc.

390 Oak Ave., Suite A

Carlsbad, CA 92008

Nuk brush Use with or without food to help kids become less defensive in the mouth. Available from Toys "R" Us or
The Equipment Shop
P.O. Box 33
Bedford, MA 01730

Sound Bites This novelty toy has a useful application. These are lollipops that make sounds inside the mouth.

Straws Drinking through a straw helps to strengthen and coordinate lip closure and sucking. Look for different straws— fat, skinny, smooth, or with ridges. These make drinking more fun and strengthen muscles around the lips.

For kids who are not quite ready to suck liquids through a straw, there are cup-straw combinations that allow an adult to squeeze a liquid into a child's mouth through a tube/straw.

The Honey Bear, with a tube, and a straw cup are examples. Both are available from catalogs (such as *Mealtimes* from New Visions) that offer eating aids. See the list of such catalogs in chapter 7, "Making Food Desirable."

Stuffed Toys or Cloths Lightly wipe the face with different textures, going from smooth to nubby.

Vibrators These provide more intense stimulation to a child's face and mouth and are best used after consulting with a therapist. Do not use them without first preparing your child. Help a child become comfortable with the vibration in stages. Go slowly with using such a device and allow your child to become comfortable with this new sensation.

There's a wide range of these, including star-shaped pacifiers or teething rings that vibrate when a child bites down. These are often found in department stores such as Target.

For the outside of the face, vibrators now come in fanciful shapes, like alligators or characters such as Casper or Ellie. These are available from the *Abilitations* catalog or www.abilitations.com.

Before these were available, therapists adapted everyday items such as the handles of electric toothbrushes.

Any of these vibrators can be used to massage a child's cheeks and the outside of the mouth. They help children relax and enjoy sensations in their mouths.

Young children vary in how quickly they gain feeding skills, both in terms of handling more difficult foods and in their ability to begin self-feeding. Keep the act of eating a positive experience for you and your child by giving your child the time he needs to acquire these new skills.

Do

- Be aware of how your child responds to new foods. Sometimes a simple change such as introducing new foods more slowly improves her willingness to try them.
- Model how to bite and chew new foods.
- Try non-food activities to strengthen mouth muscles.
- Encourage your child to self-feed.
- Look at your child's play skills to gauge his ability to self-feed.

Don't

- Use age as the sole guide to determine your child's readiness to eat more difficult foods.

- Force your child to eat foods he can't handle. Instead, prod gently and persistently.
- Expect your child to learn how to bite and chew without an occasional gag.
- Worry that your child won't be able to learn how to eat. Some children just need more time than others.

Fussy Babies

If a child has a problem with eating, a question worth asking is, When did the problem start? The answer may hold a key to a solution.

Babies enter the world hardwired to eat. For many, the first eating experience, sucking milk, is relatively problem-free.

When babies struggle with eating from day one, there's usually an underlying physical condition. Even so, most babies adjust and outgrow their problems. Those who don't may need tests, medications, special formulas, or visits with specialists, especially if growth is not on schedule.

The situation is different when feeding problems start later. Older babies, taking their first steps toward independence, often begin by trying to control their eating. This is common. In fact, most feeding problems begin between the ages of nine and eighteen months, and involve issues around self-feeding.

This chapter covers general information to help babies eat better, common feeding challenges, perspectives on babies with tube feedings, and, last, research on helping babies broaden the variety of foods that they enjoy.

Foundations

When feeding your baby, keep three fundamental truths in mind:

- Babies eat better if they learn to recognize the sensations of hunger and satiety.
- Babies eat better if you respond to their cues.
- Babies eat better when they are actively involved.

BUILDING HUNGER AWARENESS

To first-time parents it may seem as though a newborn, when awake, is always feeding. In fact, newborns need lots of small feedings, sometimes twelve or more a day. At this early stage, babies are simultaneously learning how to suck efficiently and gearing up for a growth spurt.

This means that waiting for a hunger cry may mean waiting too long. A newborn who is ready to eat might squirm, put his hands into his mouth, make sucking noises, or generally look more alert. With newborns, it's important to respond to these early signs of hunger. It helps to establish trust and keeps an infant content and less anxious about feeding. Generally, tuning in to your baby's signs of hunger is the best approach with newborns, rather than timing feedings by a clock or waiting for a baby to cry from hunger.

✕ *If your infant struggles with feeding, respond to early signs of hunger. A small infant who is overly hungry may eat less instead of more. Crying takes energy. The exertion of crying can tire out an infant and make it harder for her to settle down for a feeding.*

As babies become older and bigger, they eat more at each feeding and this sustains them for longer stretches of time. Many fall into a predictable routine, which gives parents confidence that all is well. Two things throw this schedule off:

1. **Appetite spurts** Now and then infants cry for more and seem to be insatiable. This is normal. Appetite spurts vary and, though difficult to predict, they seem most likely to happen at the ages of eight to twelve days, three to four weeks, and three months.

2. **Illness** When babies get sick, their appetites lag but soon recover. It's generally better not to worry or overreact.

✗ *Unless the doctor has concerns about your baby's growth, trust your baby's signals for hunger and satiety. Having trust in your child's ability to self-regulate calories changes the way you feed your baby. Most babies can self-regulate calories, but need encouragement and practice to develop it.*

Over time, the meaning of a baby's cry changes. By the time a baby is three months old, some parents say they recognize different cries and can differentiate the cry for hunger from other cries.

Offering a breast or bottle whenever your baby cries is a good strategy for newborns and small babies (less than sixteen pounds) or any baby that is underweight.

As babies grow older, bigger, and smarter, they are more likely to cry for reasons unrelated to hunger. After eight months, babies may begin to cry when uncomfortable or bored. If you suspect your older baby's cry is not related to hunger, you can try other comfort measures first. In some instances, offering food whenever a baby fusses suggests that food is a general all-purpose comfort and does not help a child establish a pattern of when to eat versus when not to eat. Feeding in response to hunger will help your child make a clearer connection between hunger and satiety.

✕ *When an older baby cries, give comfort and attention first and food second. If hugs, kisses, and playing with your older baby don't work, try more food or sleep. Food is the easy solution, but try to determine whether it is always the best one for your child.*

RESPOND TO YOUR BABY'S CUES

There's a surprising amount of work needed to take care of a baby, and busy, productive parents with long to-do lists feel better checking off "baby fed" after twenty rather than forty-five minutes. But babies have their own agenda. At times, newborns and young babies need coaxing and coddling to help them take in needed nourishment.

Early on, helping a baby become engaged in eating invariably slows meals down, but it is always a worthwhile goal, even when babies have feeding problems. Normally it pays off.

The cries of a newborn tend to communicate one of two messages: "I'm hungry" or "I'm uncomfortable." Because newborns are almost always hungry, it's best to feed them on demand. This means letting your baby set the pace, and following his schedule.

Later, when you introduce solid foods, adopt the same philosophy. Babies often experience their first taste of solid food between four and six months, but they vary in their readiness. Is your baby ready to eat food from a spoon? Typically, babies who are able to sit up are ready to eat food from a spoon.

Since every baby is different, you'll want to gauge your child's interest and comfort with solid foods and adjust the pace. A great way to do this is to prod your baby to give you signals. Put the spoon close to, but not actually into, your baby's mouth. Use pantomime to communicate "open your mouth." Encourage your baby to imitate. If the mouth stays shut, back off. Be friendly, smile, and try again.

Admittedly, there are babies whose mouths never seem to open for food. Try dabbing a little food on your baby's lips. Be sure to smile and then visibly lick your lips. Hopefully your baby will imitate, like the taste, and then open up for more.

✕ *Before giving up on a food, use the three-times rule. When a baby doesn't readily open his mouth for the next spoonful, parents ask, How hard should we try? A good rule is to stop after a child has refused a spoonful three consecutive times.*

Babies do more than communicate pleasure or discomfort; they learn from experience and respond to kindness. There's no doubt that your actions send a message. Even when feedings take a long time, even if no food goes into your child, remember that the back-and-forth exchange is not a waste of time. It's communicating that mealtimes are pleasant, that you are trustworthy and not determined to shove food in unexpectedly. You are willing to wait until your child is ready. Thus, most babies become *more* cooperative.

HELP YOUR BABY PARTICIPATE IN EATING

To help young babies participate in eating you often need to think less about how much food your baby eats than *how* he eats it. Wait for your baby's mouth to open for the spoon. Don't sneak food in while distracting him with a toy. Instead, draw his attention to the food and try again.

✕ *Don't use toys or games to distract babies into eating. This works at first. Babies love to play. But in the long run, shifting a baby's focus off food and onto toys or games is a mistake. Soon parents find themselves looking for bigger and better entertainment; otherwise the baby refuses to eat.*

Common pitfalls that interfere with kids being actively involved in feeding:

- feeding a baby who is asleep
- distracting a baby to get him to eat
- being too forceful

If your baby drinks from a bottle, encourage him to hold the bottle or touch it during feedings. At some point, you'll want your baby to hold his own bottle. Before this happens, he needs to have enough strength to bring his arms forward, be able to hold his hands up (and in midline), grasp his hands around the bottle, and coordinate his breathing with sucking and swallowing. All this takes practice. Make it easier for your baby to master these new skills. Start early and let him gain these skills gradually.

Early Self-Feeding

With newborns and young babies, parents control mealtimes. Around nine months the control gradually shifts as babies make their first moves toward independence. You can avoid problems by planning ahead. Encourage your child to actively participate in eating.

Even though Sam had always been a great eater, at ten months, his mother, Sheila, noticed a change in her son. When she offered Sam a spoonful of peas, he turned his head. After a second try, Sheila mumbled, "Okay, enough peas." Because Sam hadn't eaten much, she tried a spoonful of peaches. Again, he turned his head. Sheila wondered, Should I stop?

Instead of giving up, she went to the refrigerator for yogurt. In that moment of freedom, Sam grabbed the spoon.

Sheila knew Sam would make a mess. Still, she understood that her son was bright, curious, and beginning to understand cause and effect. When he pressed the buttons on his busy box or other toys, things happened: bells rang, music played or, lights blinked.

Sheila decided to let Sam keep the spoon. As expected, her adorable but clumsy son spilled peaches on himself, but he ate the yogurt, and the meal ended happily.

Despite the mess, Sheila made a good decision to let Sam keep the spoon. It kept his focus on eating. Likewise, another strategy would be to give Sam small pieces of food he could pick up with his fingers.

Older babies are driven to explore and make sense of the world. Mealtimes are not only about food; they offer opportunities to learn, explore, grow, and become self-reliant. While self-feeding offers all these benefits for kids, it tends to be a hassle for parents.

Parents realize that there are potholes in the road to independence. The early stage of self-feeding is best described as "feeding the floor." There is a big gap between what kids *can* do and what they *want* to do.

To make the early stage of self-feeding easier, plan ahead. Graham crackers or dry cereals are classic choices—easy for kids to pick up and eat and easy for parents to sweep away. Here are some strategies for less messy self-feeding:

- Add dry baby cereal to yogurt, applesauce, and other baby foods, especially those that are watery. This helps food stick to the spoon.
- Use a spoon with a perforated bowl. The holes help food stick to the spoon.
- Look for a baby spoon with a thick handle, which is easier for a small hand to hold. For more ideas on easy-to-hold feeding gear, read chapter 7, "Making Food Desirable."

- Feed your child in a high chair. This limits the mess and gets a child into a good habit.
- Spear a banana chunk onto a wooden Popsicle stick and your child will find it is easier to hold and more fun to eat.
- Take advantage of plastic floor mats, wipeable bibs, shirt-off eating, or a queen-size sheet you can throw in the washer.

Facing Challenges

Because babies are born with immature digestive, nervous, and urinary systems, early feeding problems are common. Nonetheless, few parents are ready for a baby who doesn't eat well. All feeding problems—whether minor or major—are stressful.

Even though most feeding problems with babies go away without interventions, there are problems that linger or are more worrisome. Because each child's situation is unique, seek specialized help that focuses on your child's needs. The following section discusses common problems related to sucking, digestion, growth, sleep, and feeding tubes. Some of these topics are also discussed elsewhere in this book.

KIDS AT RISK

In one survey, researchers interviewed parents of young children with eating problems and found that many had one of the following:

low birth weight
prematurity
distress during feeding in the first six months of life
regular or frequent vomiting

SOURCE: *Archives of Disease in Childhood*, October 1996, pp. 75, 304–8 (interview data on severe behavioral eating difficulties in young children).

SUCKING

In order for babies to suck effectively they need to feel comfortable and relaxed. They also need to coordinate sucking with breathing and swallowing. Signs that sucking is not easy for your baby:

- **Too many breaks** Lots of starts and stops during feedings usually mean longer feedings and that your baby may not be able to take in the recommended amount of breast milk or formula.
- **Trouble settling down** Some babies are easily distracted and need help to relax and feel comfortable while feeding.

Naturally, finding a solution involves some trial and error and possibly seeking the advice of a specialist who can watch your baby while he is feeding. Common recommendations:

- **Limit distractions.**
  Notice whether noise or light levels distract your baby while eating. Some babies find it easier to suck when noise or light levels are low.

- **Help your baby relax during feedings.**
  Rocking and swaddling are traditional techniques used to soothe babies. Experiment with swaddling before and during feedings. Try rocking your baby before feedings.

- **Look at your baby's position.**
  You may find that changing the way you hold your baby during feedings helps. If you are not breast-feeding, hold your baby up as though you were and support the neck so that your baby's chin is tucked forward toward his chest. You

may also want to support your baby's arms so that they are forward rather than rolled back. These are general suggestions. Depending on your baby's body, a therapist might recommend other changes, such as using an angled bottle, pillows for extra support, or bringing one arm forward initially.

- **Experiment with nipples.**
Breast-fed babies who use bottles as a supplement sometimes experience nipple confusion. Using round nipples with a broad base tends to encourage similar tongue and jaw movements as feeding at the breast. Specific brands to try include the Avent Newborn Slow Flow, the Playtex Natural Shape or Natural Latch, and the Evenflo Ultra or Elite.

When choosing a nipple for an exclusively bottle-fed baby, expect to find nipples that vary in size, stiffness, and shape.

Size: In order for a nipple to fit comfortably in your baby's mouth, the size needs to be in proportion to your child's body. A six-pound newborn needs a smaller nipple than a twenty-five-pound one-year-old.

Stiffness: Among the different styles of nipples, you'll notice that some are labeled slow-flow, medium-flow, or fast-flow. Most fast-flow nipples are softer, making it easier to suck through. Normally the goal is to use a nipple that is hard enough to make a baby work the mouth muscles yet soft enough to ensure that he takes in the needed volume.

Shape: If you have experimented with different-shaped nipples and none seems adequate, you'll want to seek the

advice of a specialist. In addition to all the shapes normally available, there are specialized, harder-to-find
nipples that help some babies suck more efficiently. The
nipple with the best shape for your baby will depend on
the anatomy of his mouth as well as the maturity of his
sucking skills. This is best determined by someone with
a trained eye, typically a speech therapist who has experience with feeding.

DIGESTION

Parents with young babies often deal with problems related to
gas, colic, or spitting up. Simple remedies may be worth a try.

Gas

Gas is a normal part of digestion. Don't be concerned unless it
makes your baby uncomfortable. Possible remedies include over-
the-counter Mylicon drops.

- **For breast-fed babies:**
  If you are breast-feeding and have a generous supply, try giving just one breast at each feeding. The idea is that your baby
  may be getting more foremilk, which is higher in lactose, too
  much of which causes gas.

  Although the mother's diet is not the most likely cause, in
  some cases omitting cow's milk, soy, caffeine, eggs, or peanuts
  helps.

- **For formula-fed babies:**
  Swallowed air is more often to blame than the formula. Try
  keeping the bottle tilted up so that the nipple is full while
  your baby is feeding and burp him regularly.

Colic

Although the cause is unknown, colicky babies have distended bellies, which might be caused by gas being formed during digestion or air being swallowed. In addition to burping more often, the remedies normally suggested are the same as those used to help babies suck (see page 66). Even though colic is stressful, most babies grow adequately and their symptoms improve by the time they are four to five months old.

Spitting Up (Reflux)

Spitting up is quite common in babies. It often improves when babies begin to sit up or crawl and most babies outgrow it by their first birthday. One simple remedy is to give a baby more support during feedings by holding her so that her trunk is elongated and not slumped. The idea is that being slumped increases pressure in the abdomen and makes it easier for fluid in the stomach to move upward into a baby's throat and mouth. For the same reason, avoid laying a baby down too soon after a feeding.

There's more detailed information on reflux in chapter 11, "Food Allergies and Digestion Problems."

GROWTH

Shortly after birth, newborns lose weight as they adjust to life outside the womb. Within one or two weeks they begin to grow rapidly, and by four to six months they have doubled their birth weight. To ensure that a baby's early growth is progressing on schedule, many pediatricians monitor growth closely during the first six months of life. This enables them to pick up on any problems that might arise. Even though breast milk is the best choice for the majority of babies, during this early phase of life, formula-fed babies typically gain weight faster than breast-fed babies.

To maintain adequate growth, some babies need extra calories, and a supplement or special formula may be recommended. There are commercial fortifiers designed to be added to breast milk (which is usually pumped). Normally, baby formulas provide twenty calories per ounce. Although formulas can be concentrated to increase calories, there is a potential for serious complications and it should *never* be done without medical supervision.

SLEEPING

Not all babies get off to a good start with sleeping. Their parents survive the months of sleep deprivation, but only a few do it happily. To improve your baby's sleep pattern, consider two links with their eating habits.

Body Size

Initially, infants are too small to sleep a long stretch without feeding. Their stomachs do not hold enough to fuel their bodies for more than a few hours. But as the months go by and babies grow bigger, they don't need to be fed as often. Normally, babies need to weigh at least sixteen pounds before they sleep through the night.

✕ *Don't expect a newborn to sleep through the night. Newborns need special care. Encouraging a baby to sleep through the night is a worthwhile goal for older babies, but not for newborns. If a newborn sleeps four hours or more without fussing to be fed, call the pediatrician for advice. A general rule of thumb is that infants who weigh less than fifteen pounds need at least one nighttime feeding.*

Eating and Sleeping

Infants often sleep well after a good feeding and often doze off while sucking. But as babies grow older, routines around sleeping and eating change. That is, they need to change if parents want to help babies learn how to fall asleep on their own. Typically that means learning how to fall asleep so that dozing off does not always coincide with being fed, held, or rocked. Sleep experts often suggest putting babies in the crib while sleepy but not yet fully asleep.

The National Sleep Foundation offers information online about sleep patterns in babies and ideas on how to help a baby sleep well. Their Web site is www.sleepfoundation.org. They offer a free brochure, *Sleep, Your Baby and You*. You can order it by calling 1-866-565-2229. For a $1.00 postage and handling fee you can order the brochure and a sleep sheet, "Children and Sleep: Helping Your Child Develop Healthy Sleep Habits." Mail to

Department PS
National Sleep Foundation
1522 K Street, NW, Suite 500
Washington, DC 20005

If your baby is sick and resists eating, you may be tempted to feed him while he sleeps. This is not usually recommended. A baby who is asleep during a feeding will find it harder to associate hunger with the satisfaction of eating. Making this association is a critical step in the process of learning to self-regulate calories.

FEEDING TUBES

Undoubtedly, feeding tubes bring another layer of complexity to feeding, yet the same principles apply. Reading your child's cues and encouraging him to participate will make a difference in how he experiences food.

Babies who can't eat by mouth and are fed through feeding

tubes will eat better later if they are given a pacifier or other oral experiences to stimulate the mouth during feedings. Again, this helps a child to associate sensations in the mouth with satiety— an important first step in learning to eat by mouth.

When it's time to begin eating food by mouth, it's still important to encourage a child to *want* to eat. This is one of the toughest goals parents face when weaning a child off a feeding tube. Yet trying to understand a child's needs and personality can enable parents to dream up unique ways to motivate a child to eat. I witnessed one child's amazing and inspiring transition off tube feeding.

As a newborn, Sammy had significant medical problems, which meant that it wasn't safe for him to take food or formula by mouth. Instead he was fed through a feeding tube that went into his stomach.

Two surgeries and six months later, the doctor gave the approval for Sammy to begin eating by mouth. He promised that when Sammy ate well and often enough, he would remove the feeding tube. Like most parents, Sammy's mom, Wendy, was thrilled and determined to make this happen as soon as possible.

To help him learn to eat by mouth, Wendy took seven-month-old Sammy to see a feeding specialist. In addition to performing oral-motor exercises to prepare his mouth, she and the therapist made the sessions fun while gently and playfully prodding Sammy to do more. But it was a slow process, and Sammy still didn't eat more than a few licks, sips, or spoonfuls of anything.

Along the way, there were also some unavoidable missed appointments. Yet Sammy's mom was determined to help him learn to eat by mouth. But she also realized that if she forced him to eat, he would resist. She thought about ways to motivate Sammy. One thing was obvious to her: he was a very social baby who loved being around people.

Even though he didn't eat, once a day she included her son at the dinner table, hoping he would take food. Normally he refused. One day she decided to change her approach. She put Sammy in his high chair a few feet away from the dinner table. Once Sammy realized that everyone else was eating dinner, he fussed. He *wanted* to join everyone at the table. Once there, he wanted to join the group activity: eating.

This was a turning point for Sammy. Although the move to eating by mouth was slow at the beginning, his mom felt that the patience had paid off. By the time he was fourteen months old, Sammy was eating and drinking by mouth.

Considering Sammy's complex medical needs, he made remarkable progress transitioning off tube feeding. I believe that Sammy's age and his mother's ability to balance her own determination with his needs and personality made the difference.

Influencing Your Baby's Taste

Can parents prime children's taste buds to like vegetables? This question tends to come up after a baby starts cereal and is ready to try new foods.

Parents often are told to give vegetables before fruit. This strategy is based on the theory that if sweet-flavored fruits are given first, it heightens a baby's preference for sweets. Alas, researchers report that there's no scientific evidence to support this.

Yet parents suspect there must be *something* they can do to help their baby develop a taste for healthy foods. After all, while they may be in the minority, kids who like vegetables and other healthy foods do exist.

For more than twenty years, Julie Mennella from Philadelphia's Monell Chemical Senses Center has done research exploring when and how babies develop flavor preferences. An obvious first question involves timing: When do babies first develop these preferences? Studies in animals and humans suggest that it could begin in the womb—fetuses experience chemosensory stimulation through amniotic fluid, which has both odor and flavor.

Considering this, could a woman's food choices while pregnant influence her unborn baby's taste preferences? According to at least one small study, the answer is yes. Mennella asked mothers-to-be to drink carrot juice and found that months later their babies demonstrated a stronger liking for carrot-flavored cereal.

Unlike formula, which provides one constant taste experience, the flavor of breast milk changes from one day to the next, depending on the foods a mother eats. Researchers have speculated that there could be a biological reason; maybe this is nature's way of gradually introducing babies to the flavors and spices that they will soon experience firsthand.

Formal studies show that breast-fed infants are more willing to try a new vegetable than those who are formula-fed. Although Mennella cites the benefits of breast-feeding, she has also done re-

---

THE CARROT JUICE STUDY

Julie Mennella, a behavioral scientist with the Monell Center in Philadelphia, divided forty-six pregnant women into three groups. The first group drank carrot juice during the last trimester of pregnancy and switched to water when breast-feeding. The second group did the opposite, and the third group drank only water throughout. Months later, all the babies ate cereal that was mixed with water one day and carrot juice the next. In the end, the infants from the first two groups—those exposed to the carrot flavor through amniotic fluid or breast-feeding—ate three times more carrot-flavored cereal than the infants whose mothers drank only water.

search with formula-fed babies, again showing that they too benefit from experiencing varied food flavors.

Early on, breast milk is the safest way to increase the variety of flavors a baby experiences. But later, all babies expand flavor experiences with the introduction of food.

When a group of formula-fed infants were ready to start solid food, some were given a single new vegetable (potatoes or carrots) while others were given several new vegetables. The first time chicken was offered, those given a variety of vegetables (peas, potatoes, and squash) ate more chicken than the babies who had eaten only one vegetable—potatoes. They also ate more carrots than the potatoes-only group, even though they had never tasted carrots before.

✕ *Help your baby enjoy food by experiencing different food flavors. When your baby begins to eat solid foods, avoid mixing them together. Instead let your baby experience each new flavor separately. This makes eating more interesting and helps your baby enjoy a variety of food flavors.*

Mennella has taken the idea a step further to explore the limits of when babies are open to new flavors and, as parents may suspect, when this ends. For medical reasons, babies sometimes need specialized formulas that taste unpleasant, or downright vile, to most adults. Yet babies don't seem to mind the bitter taste. That is, they don't mind if the formula is introduced early—before four months of age. Up to this age, there's usually no problem with a baby accepting a formula, regardless of the flavor.

Research suggests that the best way to increase the variety of foods kids eat is to expose them to a variety of food flavors early on. The focus should be on trying new foods rather than eating large amounts. Babies benefit from a taste here and there.

Although they do show flavor preferences early, parents may need to try and try again.

✕ *If a baby refuses to eat a food the first time, don't give up. Babies need time to recognize and enjoy new food flavors. Researchers have found that sometimes babies need to try a food eight to ten times before they begin to enjoy it.*

Babies eventually grow older and parents can't help but wonder whether or not early food experiences have a lasting effect. National food studies suggest that, as a group, children make healthier food choices when they are younger. Some speculate that this is due to parents controlling the foods available.

As kids grow, the number of influences on their food choices expands. For better or worse, there's always the possibility that a social experience, a teacher, a friend, or an ad will spark a change in a child's list of desirable foods. Over time, it becomes harder to isolate any one influence consistently affecting a majority of children. And, as everyone knows, older children do not always follow an adult's advice in making food choices. Yet one small study offers hope.

Researchers looked at the food choices of seventy children during infancy and then again six to eight years later. They found connections between early food exposures and the choices the children made a few years later. Vegetable variety in the school-age children was related to the mother's vegetable preferences early on. Breast-feeding duration and either early fruit variety or early fruit exposure influenced fruit variety for the school-age children.

This study is somewhat unusual in that it followed the same group of children over a number of years. But the results, while limited, are encouraging and suggest that parents do have a positive influence on their children's food choices.

WHAT IS TASTE?

We experience "flavor" through two senses: smell and taste. When we think of savoring food flavors, we imagine the taste buds on our tongues as key. This is only partially true. Taste receptors in the mouth register a small number of primary tastes of sweet, salty, bitter, sour, and "umami" (savory). Taste cells appear in the human fetus at about fourteen weeks. And scientists believe that basic taste preferences are hardwired into humans.

Our ability to taste food is strongly affected by smell, which is a much more complicated mechanism. There are potentially thousands of different classes of odor stimuli. Compared to taste, our sense of smell is both more complex and more soft-wired. That is, our smell preferences are influenced by early exposure. The smells we like as adults are linked to the odors we experienced while young. Experts on odor preferences find patterns based on early smell experiences. For example, those who were babies during the era when Johnson's baby powder was standard choice tend to prefer certain aromas over those who as babies were exposed to other odors.

If we want to influence which food flavors our kids are likely to prefer as they grow older, allowing them to smell healthy foods is probably a good bet!

While it seems that babies eat instinctively, psychologists describe eating as a *learned* behavior shaped by early experiences. Although you may not be able to control all of your baby's feeding problems, as you work through the difficulties, remember to be sensitive to your baby's cues and encourage her to give you signals. The give-and-take teaches your baby to trust you.

This is a good foundation for the next stage. As your baby grows into a toddler, you'll face new challenges. Toddlers typically don't need much encouragement to give signals for what they want or don't want. For this stage you'll need to change gears and begin setting limits on *what* and *how* your child eats. This usually goes more smoothly when there's a bond of trust between you.

BASIC REMINDERS WHEN FEEDING BABIES

Do
- Feed newborns on demand and at the first sign of hunger.
- Try to distinguish a hunger cry from a cry for attention or sleep.
- Experiment with nipples on bottles or positioning if your baby tires easily while sucking.
- Take your time with early spoon-feeding and respond to your baby's signals. Stop after your baby gives three consecutive signals that he doesn't want any more.
- Encourage independence as it emerges.
- Provide mouth stimulation for babies fed with tubes.

Don't
- Mix all your baby's food together into one big mush. Let her experience individual food flavors.
- Feed babies while they are asleep.
- Use food to comfort babies who are upset but not hungry. Don't automatically feed an older baby every time he cries.
- Use physical force to feed.

Fussy Toddlers and Preschoolers

Even though picky eaters often make poor food choices, most of them are healthy, inquisitive, and inclined to test limits. This is a potentially volatile combination!

When a child does not eat as expected, loving parents can find themselves seriously distressed. Countless parents lose sleep, and in some families, a picky eater tips the balance of family harmony into a downward free fall.

All this fretting over food is unfortunate because finicky eating is normal behavior for toddlers. Like teething and other parts of growing up, although unpleasant, it is largely unavoidable. There are biological and developmental forces that drive the change in a young child's appetite.

Even though picky eating is a passing phase for most children, there are exceptions. Some picky eaters have more complex needs. This is especially true when a child is not gaining weight or not eating like other children of the same age. Regardless of the cause, a better understanding of a child's developmental needs offers insights into how to best handle food refusals.

Shifting Needs

Richard Canfield, professor of human development at Cornell University, describes the behavior change in young children as so fundamental and profound that he thinks of children at each new stage as a different species. After the age of six months, there's a rapid and drastic change in mealtime dynamics. In less than a year, babies move from total dependence on parents to self-feeding. Babies rarely refuse food, while toddlers delight in saying no to just about everything.

Canfield describes toddlers as "motors without pilots." This helps explain why mealtimes with toddlers are so challenging. Preschoolers are more open to new experiences, and sometimes this includes food. As a child moves from one developmental stage to the next, the strategies needed to achieve happier mealtimes change.

SELF-FEEDING

Young toddlers from one to two years old still need considerably more practice before they master self-feeding. Despite their limited skills, most toddlers *want* to feed themselves. Babies begin grabbing the spoon long before they develop the coordination to successfully use it—typically at around eighteen months. Like walking and talking, mastering basic food skills takes practice. First there's the problem of getting food into the mouth. Initially, this means developing a reliably firm and coordinated grip on bottles and/or cups. Toddlers can usually drink from a bottle or cup without help. First they learn to hold it with both hands and later with one. The next challenge is solid foods.

Most one-year-olds can pick up food with their fingers and normally prefer to eat finger foods. But from time to time they will want to use a spoon. This takes months of practice. Professionals focus on technical details: Does the child lift the elbow and flex the wrist as the spoon reaches the mouth? Parents focus on how much food they need to clean off the child, tray, and floor. Normally kids don't use a spoon without spilling some food until age two. Luckily, the learning curve for using a fork is faster and less messy.

Once food reaches the mouth, there's still more to learn. Even after children have advanced to eating table foods, they still need to practice biting, chewing, and swallowing. Young children benefit by chewing tougher foods, but most refuse to eat anything that takes too much effort. This is why toddlers often resist eating meats and other tough, chewy foods. There's also the problem that not all foods are safe for young children to eat—especially hard foods such as nuts, raw carrots, and hard candies. None of these is recommended for children under the age of three.

✕ *Keep an eye on your child when he eats. Eating while talking, laughing, or moving about makes even familiar foods risky. The risk of choking is greatest for kids under the age of two. The coordination of chewing with swallowing is not fully developed until the age of eight.*

TODDLER BEHAVIOR

With toddlers, the mechanics of *how* to eat become less important. At this age, the big question becomes, Does the child *want* to eat? Too often, the answer is no, and this, combined with a child's need to become independent, underlies many problems parents face. Never ask a toddler if he wants to eat. Simply announce that it is time to eat.

When the parents' sole focus is on getting a child to eat healthy foods without recognizing a toddler's natural need for independence, mealtime battles are sure to escalate. If you don't want your child to eat junk foods, keep them out of the house. This is not a good age to teach self-restraint.

Toddlers need you to ignore some of their nonsensical food choices and to set limits. It's tricky to give toddlers some control but not too much. And regardless of what parents do or don't do, toddlers are known to be difficult. Expect to face any of the following:

- **Fussy preferences**
  Toddlers can be demanding. Some will fuss about foods touching, or broken crackers or cookies. They may insist on using a special cup. You can try to accommodate such eccentricities, but don't go overboard. When a toddler makes demands that are too difficult for you to provide, just say so. Be nice but firm.

- **Slow eating**
  Toddlers often have immature biting and chewing skills and may need extra time. As long as a toddler wants to eat, you should give him the time he needs. Just make sure that he is actually eating and not being distracted by television, siblings, or toys.

- **Refusal to sit in a high chair**
  It's good to insist that if a child wants to eat she must sit in the high chair. At some point many toddlers scream to move out. A booster seat at the table is a good next step. Sometimes the type of high chair or the associations with it make a difference. One set of twins used their high chairs well past their third birthday without a fuss. They easily climbed in and out of their heavy wooden high chairs for breakfast, and when they wanted to use Play-Doh or other "messy" projects.

- **Short-order cooking**
  Encourage a toddler to make food choices. When possible, offer two options: "Do you want an apple or an orange?" But when several foods are available and a toddler refuses, don't offer a new food. This teaches children that if they say no to food they may get something better.

  One mother complained that following this suggestion was especially hard to do at dinner. "If I give her choices and she won't eat, I can't believe she won't wake up early starving." Giving her daughter milk as part of her bedtime routine helped her not to worry.

- **Nighttime feedings**
  Toddlers are generally big enough and old enough to sleep through the night. One reason they don't is habit. The simple solution is to try to gradually stop feeding calorie-containing foods or beverages during the night. Instead of giving milk, slowly change to water.

- **Food throwing**
  Assume that a child who throws food does not want to eat. Matter-of-factly and as soon as possible, pick up the food and toss it into the trash, saying "Bye-bye, food." Avoid getting visibly angry or upset. If you are worried that your child will be hungry and cranky, you can move the next meal or snack to an earlier time.

The potential tangles with a toddler over food are endless. Gina stands in front of a cabinet screaming for pretzels. Audrey refuses to eat homemade chicken nuggets. The twins, Kyle and Kelsey, both want the same blue cup.

Whatever the issue, one simple solution is to redirect a child's attention to something else. Instead of screaming back, "No, you can't have the cup with the dragons," change the subject: "Oh, look, it's almost one o'clock, we need to get ready for _____." With a little practice, you'll be amazed at how effectively you can redirect your child's attention.

When Gina stood screaming in front of the kitchen cabinet filled with snack foods, her mother discovered that she could divert Gina's attention by turning on the water faucet and letting Gina play in the sink. This seemed better, but not much. Her mother realized she was trading one problem for another.

After thinking it over, she tried a new strategy. She put away one of Gina's favorite toys. When she needed to redirect her daughter's attention, she took out the favorite toy. This worked so well that she eventually did it with three different toys and rotated them.

Mealtimes are easier when a toddler feeds himself. This keeps him busy and appropriately focused on food. Not all toddlers willingly feed themselves. Sometimes young children *want* or *need* parents to help. The timetable for self-feeding may be different for

- triplets or twins who compete for parent attention.
- preemies or other children with special needs.
- children in homes with cultural traditions that don't emphasize independence.

If your toddler wants to be fed, you'll need to think through how much help to give and when to stop. Young children want help for emotional as well as developmental reasons. When parents ask my advice, I always consider the following:

- How well can the child feed himself?
- Why does he want help?

Donna thought through these questions when her son Scott asked for help at meals. Four-year-old Scott regressed after the arrival of a new baby brother. He wanted his mother to feed him too. Donna encouraged Scott to be a "big boy" and feed himself but made one exception. She fed him spaghetti, which was more difficult for him to manage. This small indulgence helped Scott feel special. To avoid constant battles, Donna made it clear that spaghetti was the only food she would feed him.

PRESCHOOLER BEHAVIOR

Defiant toddlers often mellow as their awareness of the world grows. They begin to see the possibility of adults as allies. Preschoolers are still likely to say no to new foods, but less so than toddlers.

Although the need for independence continues and the pitfalls for gaining attention through food remain, preschoolers are less impulsive and can follow instructions. These changes give parents more options around food. Preschoolers

- enjoy touching, looking at, and smelling food. If you talk about a food, go shopping, or cook together, the odds go up that it will be eaten or at least tasted.
- ask questions and want to know more about the world. That curiosity can spill over to food.
- need to show that they can do things by themselves. Asking preschoolers to help set the table or cook makes meals more appealing.
- are more comfortable in unfamiliar places. At this stage, it becomes easier to take them to malls, restaurants, and other places that offer new foods.

HUNGER AWARENESS IN TODDLERS AND PRESCHOOLERS

For toddlers, eating is noticeably less automatic than it is for babies. Toddlers regularly ignore opportunities to eat, even when it seems obvious that they should be hungry. Bigger bodies and slower growth rates help them to go for surprisingly long periods without food. But these are not the only reasons why toddlers refuse food. As they gain social awareness, toddlers learn to use food to gain attention. Also, their burgeoning interest in exploring the outside world makes it harder for them to tune in to the subtle feelings of hunger.

Helping toddlers recognize hunger is challenging. Constantly offering food does not help. In fact, spacing out meals and snacks so that they are two or more hours apart allows them to experience mild hunger and the satisfaction from eating. Limiting constant drinking of juice or milk also helps. The constant sipping of calorie-laden drinks dulls appetite signals, causing some children to overeat and others to undereat.

For preschoolers and older children, pointing out tummy growls, thirst, and other signals our bodies provide helps them to recognize internal cues for eating. This is the goal.

Be a model. Talk about being hungry or full. Don't binge-eat or demonstrate out-of-control eating. Ask a toddler questions such as "Are you hungry?"; "Is your tummy empty?"; "Time to fill your tummy?"

One study involving three- and four-year-olds focused on these techniques. Kids learned about hunger and satiety through a video (*Winnie the Pooh and the Honey Tree*), and by watching a skit that highlighted hunger (rumbling in the stomach), eating to fullness (stomach extension and fullness), and the signals associated with overeating (stomach distension and discomfort). They also learned about body parts associated with eating, such as the mouth, stomach, and esophagus. Ideas of hunger, fullness, and overeating were also discussed through doll play using dolls that had tummies that were visible. In the end, the study demonstrated that three- and four-year-olds could improve their ability to self-regulate calories.

Recognizing what hunger feels like helps us to eat in response to internal cues—cues that the body needs more fuel. Unfortunately, too few adults eat in response to internal cues; far too often adults eat in response to external cues.

Experts caution parents to resist instructing kids to eat according to external signals such as the time of day or food left on a plate. Doing this makes it harder for kids to tune in to their own body signals of hunger or fullness.

Parents can help kids focus on internal hunger signals and improve their ability to self-regulate calories. Here are some guidelines:

BASIC REMINDERS WHEN FEEDING TODDLERS

Do
- Encourage self-feeding.
- Be a good role model and eat with your child.
- Give small portions and encourage your child to ask for more.
- Talk about being hungry or full.

Don't
- Ignore food throwing. This is a sign your child no longer wants to eat.
- Let your child see binge- or out-of-control eating.
- Insist that your child clean the plate.
- Use food as a reward, punishment, or bribe.

BASIC REMINDERS WHEN FEEDING PRESCHOOLERS

Do

- Talk about hunger, fullness, and overeating. Relate this to physical signs of comfort and discomfort. For example: "My stomach is empty. I'm hungry."
- Ask questions that help kids tune in to their internal body signals: "Are you hungry?"; "Is your tummy full?"; "Is your tummy empty?"; "Is your tummy growling?"
- Watch a food-related video, such as *Winnie the Pooh and the Honey Tree,* and talk about eating and fullness.
- Offer wholesome foods you want your child to eat.
- Encourage your child to decide *if* or *how much* to eat.

Don't

- Restrict food in obvious ways that lead to constant battles.
- Give constant directives on what your child should or should not eat.
- Allow your child to eat on the go.
- Make it a habit to eat while watching television.

PART

II

How Much Nutrition Is Enough?

National food surveys have found that many children do not meet the recommendations for specific nutrients, such as calcium, iron, and zinc. What should concerned parents do?

According to social scientists, completely controlling what your child does or doesn't eat isn't the answer. In the long run, children really need to *want* to eat wholesome foods and to develop internal control over *how much* to eat. Interestingly, national surveys show that children under the age of five meet more of the nutrition recommendations than older children do. Researchers have speculated that this is because parents provide food for younger children while older children make more of their own food choices.

To help your child make healthy foods choices on their own, you need to plan ahead.

✗ *Expect your child to refuse some of the foods you offer.* Your job as a parent is to offer a balanced variety of wholesome foods and allow your child to decide *which* foods to eat and how much. *Encourage your child to eat healthy foods by being a good example and by doing what you can to make meals pleasant.*

✕ *Keep a watchful eye on the foods your child eats.* When it comes to *influencing your child's food choices, think of yourself as a coach rather than a director. Notice what foods your child eats and when. If you notice any patterns, use that insight to plan the foods you offer. To do so, you'll need to know the basic food recommendations for children.*

Keeping it Simple

Day by day, lots of children don't eat a balanced variety of foods, but fortunately, over the stretch of a week or so, their choices tend to balance out. By offering basic foods regularly, your kids can make up what they missed one day on another day.

At each meal, offer three to four different foods. Be sure to include a protein (milk or meat group), a fruit or vegetable, and a grain. This ensures a reasonable balance, gives a child choices, and limits the tendency to offer one food after another, which encourages pickiness. The serving sizes are a guide for the amount to offer. If a child wants more, give it.

How Much Is Enough?

Picky eaters can be so picky that they refuse every possible food in one of the basic food groups, leaving parents baffled and wondering just how much calcium, protein, and other nutrients their child needs. Keep in mind that determining exact nutrition needs is difficult.

When a child doesn't take in the recommended amount of calcium, the body tries to compensate by absorbing more efficiently. When a child eats foods with iron, the amount absorbed varies.

Group Number of Servings Daily Total	Major Nutrients	Foods	Serving Sizes 1–3 years	4–5 years
Meats/Beans 2–4 servings 1.5–3 oz./day	Protein Iron Zinc	Poultry, Meat, Fish	2 tbsp	1–1½ oz.
		Beans, Tofu, Hummus	2–4 tbsp	⅓ cup
		Eggs	½	1
		Peanut butter		2 Tbsp
Milk 3–4 servings 2 cups/day	Calcium Protein Vitamins D and E	Milk/yogurt	4–6 oz.	4–6 oz.
		Natural cheese	¾ oz.	¾ oz.
		Processed cheese	1 oz.	1 oz.
Fruits and Vegetables 4–6 servings 1½–2 cups/ day	Vitamin A Vitamin C Micro-nutrients	Vitamin A *Every other day* Apricots, cantaloupe, carrots, collards, mango, pumpkin, spinach, sweet potatoes, winter squash	2–3 tbsp	¼–½ cup
		Vitamin C *Every day* Citrus fruits, kiwi, broccoli, green pepper, papaya		
Grains 4–6 servings 2–4 oz./day	B vitamins Iron (if enriched)	Rice, pasta	4–5 tbsp	½ cup
		Oatmeal, farina, grits	1–2 tbsp	3–5 tbsp
		Ready-to-eat cereals	½ cup	½ cup
		Bread, tortilla, bagels, English muffins	½ slice	1 slice
Extras	High in calories and low in nutrients	Bacon, cakes, cookies, chips, cream cheese, ketchup, doughnuts, soft drinks, syrup	No amounts recommended. Use in moderation.	

Parents should aim for the recommended amounts with the realization that these are guidelines.

CALCIUM

RECOMMENDED AMOUNTS

Age	Calcium
1–3	500 mg
4–8	800 mg
9–18	1300 mg

Two-year-old Irene refuses to drink milk or eat cheese. She is not alone. Traditionally American kids have met their calcium needs by drinking milk and eating other dairy foods. But things have changed. Over the last twenty years, kids have been drinking less milk. Some researchers speculate that as a result, kids face a greater risk for bone fractures. For strong teeth and bones, kids need calcium.

Kids who don't drink milk may struggle to get the recommended amounts of calcium. Luckily, other foods besides dairy products contain calcium—some naturally, while others, like orange juice and rice milk, are fortified.

✕ *Help make milk a habit. When kids learn to drink from a cup regularly, put milk or formula in it. Too often kids get in the habit of drinking juice/water from a cup and milk/formula from the bottle. If they associate milk only with the bottle, often when the bottle goes away, the habit of drinking milk goes with it.*

ADDING CALCIUM:
- **Dry milk powder**
  Add to mashed potatoes, macaroni and cheese, or shakes.
  Mix into batters of pancakes, muffins, and other baked goods.

- **Parmesan cheese**
  Sprinkle on pasta, soup, pizza, or casseroles.
  Put some in a shaker and encourage your child to use it.
- **Fortified Foods**
  Try one of the many calcium-fortified foods such as breakfast bars, beverages, or cereals.

CALCIUM-RICH FOODS
(approximately 300 mg each)

DAIRY

1 cup milk/yogurt	2 cups cottage cheese
1 oz. (1½ slices) cheese	½ cup ricotta (part skim)
1 cup pudding	½ cup evaporated milk

NONDAIRY

1 cup calcium-fortified soy/ rice milk	1 cup calcium-fortified orange juice
1 cup almonds	1½ cups collard greens (cooked)
1½ cups sunflower seeds	
1 cup calcium-set tofu	3 cups broccoli or kale
1 cup rhubarb	2 cups chinese cabbage (bok choy)
4 oz. salmon, canned with bones	1 cup turnip greens
2 tbsp. blackstrap molasses	5 tbsp. sesame butter (tahini)
2½ tbsp. poppy seeds	

PROTEIN

RECOMMENDED AMOUNTS

Age	Protein
1–3	16 g
4–6	24 g
7–10	28 g

Like her father, Amanda loves to eat meat. He supports her, and believes that if her body craves meat she must need it. Her mother wonders if too much can be harmful. But hundreds of kids consume double the amount of protein they need without any problem.

Amanda is four years old, an age when kids are likely to eat meat, especially if they see others enjoy it. Younger kids, namely toddlers, tend not to prefer meat, often because it requires more time and effort to chew. Yet the majority gets the protein they need through other foods—most often milk.

Milk is high in protein—which is a good thing for toddlers who don't eat meat. A toddler who drinks sixteen ounces of milk gets enough protein and calcium for the day.

PROTEIN RICH FOODS
(approximately 8 g each)

1 cup milk	1 oz. meat, fish, or chicken
1 cup yogurt	2 tbsp. peanut butter
1½ oz. American cheese	½ cup red beans
1 oz. Cheddar cheese	¼ cup sesame butter
¾ oz. Parmesan cheese	(tahini)
⅓ cup tofu	½ cup hummus
1 extra-large egg	¼ cup wheat germ

ADDING PROTEIN

- **Eggs**

    Add an extra egg to homemade foods such as pancakes, waffles, cakes, cookies, or bread. (Reduce other liquids in the recipe by 1/4 cup for each egg.)

    For kids who like soup, try the Chinese technique of whisking a beaten egg into hot soup and watch soft, thin strands of egg form.

Stir scrambled egg (with or without cheese) into hot casseroles or pasta. (To avoid salmonella food poisoning, make sure that the eggs are cooked.)

- **Peanut butter** This old standby is now a controversial food. The risks include the danger of choking for a young child who does not yet chew and swallow well. There's also the concern of an allergic reaction to peanuts. Because the incidence of peanut allergy has doubled in the last ten years, some experts suggest waiting until children are four years old before giving them peanuts. Discuss the risks and benefits with your pediatrician.

- **Wheat germ** This high-fiber food can also help with constipation.

  Stir it into hot cereals or stews.

  Sprinkle onto yogurt, pudding, or ice cream.

- **Beans** Beans, lentils, and other dried legumes are high in protein and fiber. Those who don't like them whole will often eat them in foods like hummus, which can be used as a spread or a dip.

IRON

RECOMMENDED AMOUNTS

Age	Iron
1–3	7 mg
4–8	10 mg

Iron deficiency is the most common nutritional disorder in the world. For young children, risk for iron-deficiency anemia is greatest between the ages of six months and three years.

Studies have found that kids who are anemic may score lower on intelligence tests and have poorer motor skills. Iron helps bring

---

KIDS AT GREATEST RISK FOR LOW IRON

- Low-birth-weight infants over 2 months of age
- Breast-fed babies over 4 months of age who don't eat iron-fortified foods or take a supplement
- Toddlers who drink more than 32 oz. of milk per day

---

oxygen to every cell in the body—helping brains think and muscles move. Kids who have enough iron perform better. According to researchers, the adverse affects of severe anemia can be long-lasting, affecting performance years later. Yet despite its vital importance, we need only a small amount and too much is harmful.

For most nutrients, there's no easy test to determine whether or not our bodies have the right amount, but that is not true for iron. Pediatricians normally check the iron status in young children through simple blood tests. Don't give your child an iron supplement without your doctor's approval.

Not all iron found in foods is the same. In fact, food contains two different forms of iron: heme and nonheme. Heme iron is found in meat, fish, and poultry. This is the form the human body absorbs best. Nonheme iron is found in plant foods and includes flours, grains, and cereals that are enriched or fortified. Because nonheme iron is harder for the human body to absorb, kids who don't eat meats, dairy foods, or eggs may need twice as much. Animal proteins not only provide a more efficient form of iron, they also increase the absorption of nonheme iron found in plant foods. Since the majority of Americans eat meat, standard recom-

---

HOW MUCH IS TOO MUCH IRON?

Kids under 13 should not have more than 40 mg of iron per day.

---

mendations assume that 75 percent of iron comes from heme sources.

FOODS WITH HEME IRON 3 oz. portions		FOODS WITH NONHEME IRON ½-cup portions	
chicken liver	7 mg	fortified cereals	6–12 mg
beef	3 mg	soybeans	4 mg
turkey, dark meat	2 mg	lentils	3 mg
turkey, light meat	1 mg	oatmeal (instant) fortified	2 mg
tuna	1 mg	beans	2 mg
chicken breast	1 mg	spinach	3 mg

Kids with anemia may not be able to consume enough iron from food; they may need a supplement. Some may dislike the taste. To minimize rejection, start with half the recommended dose, gradually increasing to a full dose. Also, taking the supplement in divided doses or with food may help. Foods high in vitamin C will increase iron absorption, while those high in calcium will decrease it.

Giving iron supplements

If your child refuses to take an iron supplement, try one of the following strategies:

- If your child uses a liquid supplement, mask the flavor of liquid iron supplement by mixing it with a small amount of flavored syrup such as Zarex or one of the Italian syrups used to flavor coffee drinks. (These are briefly described in chapter 8, "Food Textures and Flavors.") Mix a small amount of syrup with liquid iron in a small cup. Follow with a drink of water.

- If your child is older, eats table foods, and chews well, look for cherry-flavored chewables available in health-food stores. Discuss this with the pediatrician to make sure that the dosage matches your child's needs.

✕ *Maximize the effectiveness of supplements. If your child needs an iron supplement, maximize absorption by giving it with fruit juice high in vitamin C. At the supermarket, read labels and look for foods fortified with ferrous iron, which is better absorbed than ferric.*

FLUORIDE

RECOMMENDED AMOUNTS

Age	Fluoride
1–3	0.7 mg
4–8	1.1 mg

Fluoride, like iron, is a micronutrient. Here again, getting the right amount matters. Small amounts of fluoride make teeth stronger and more resistant to cavities. In the 1950s cities and towns across the United States began adding fluoride to the public water supply. As a result, the rate of cavities dropped.

Too much fluoride can cause fluorosis—a condition in which there are changes in bone structure and a mottling discoloration of teeth. Kids who swallow toothpaste are at risk of getting too much fluoride.

HOW MUCH IS TOO MUCH FLUORIDE?

Age	Amount per day
1–3 years	1.3 mg
4–8 years	2.2 mg
after age 9	10 mg

Generally, kids who drink tap water don't need a fluoride supplement. The amount of water a child needs to get enough fluoride depends on the amount in the water. To look up how much fluoride is in your municipal water supply, check the CDC (Centers for Disease Control) government Web site: http://apps.nccd. cdc.gov/MWF/Index.asp.

Kids who don't drink tap water, either directly or through foods made with it, may need a supplement. The amount of fluoride a child needs varies according to age and body size. Fluoride drops make it easier to give the exact amount needed by smaller, younger children. For older kids, multivitamins with fluoride are available.

✕ *Bottled water often lacks fluoride. Check the label and contact the manufacturer or bottler for information on the fluoride content. The Web site www.bottledwater.org lists companies that produce bottled water containing fluoride.*

ZINC

RECOMMENDED AMOUNTS

Age	Zinc
1–3	3 mg
4–8	5 mg

Low intake of zinc is associated with poor growth, dermatitis (skin irritation), and diarrhea.

Foods that naturally contain zinc include seafood (especially oysters), meats, and legumes. But it is also added to fortified foods such as ready-to-eat cereals.

As with iron, the absorption of zinc from different foods varies. Vegetarians may not absorb zinc as well.

ZINC IN FOODS

Food	Portion	zinc/mg
beef	1 oz.	1.5
turkey (dark meat)	1 oz.	1.3
turkey (light meat)	1 oz.	.6
Cheddar cheese	1 oz.	1.14
beans (canned)	½ cup	1
milk	1 cup	1
wheat germ	1 tbsp.	1.2
peanuts	1 oz.	.85
raisin bran	½ cup	1.75

FATS

Babies need more fat than adults do. Almost half of the calories in human milk or formula come from fat. Fat provides a concentrated form of calories for small bodies that are growing rapidly. It is also important for brain growth: 90 percent of brain growth is complete by a baby's first birthday and 95 percent by eighteen months.

As we grow older, too much fat becomes a problem, for risk of both obesity and heart disease. As a result, the amount of fat recommended drops. For children from one to three years old, the percentage of recommended calories coming from fat drops to 30 to 40 percent, while for children from ages four to eight, it drops further to 25 to 35 percent.

The amount of fat young children consume varies quite a bit. Those who like milk and cheese tend to be on the high end, while those who eat low-fat meats, fruits, and vegetables may not be getting enough, especially if they are underweight.

The timing of when to switch your child to lower-fat milk will depend on his age, weight, and family health history. Generally, you might want to substitute 2 percent milk between the ages of two and three and 1 percent milk between the ages of three and five. Ask your child's doctor when the best time is to change from whole milk to lower-fat milk.

Essential Fatty Acids

Many children do not eat foods that provide recommended amounts of essential fatty acids. Generally, kids get enough omega-6 since this is found in many commonly used vegetable oils. Often the one that is low or missing is the omega-3.

An easy way to increase this for children, especially if they don't eat fish, is to use the omega-3-enriched eggs that are now available in most supermarkets or to use cereals and other foods made with flaxseeds.

OMEGA-3 SOURCES	OMEGA-6 SOURCES
Fish oil	Corn oil
Flaxseeds or oil	Grapeseed oil
Herring	Peanut oil
Mackerel	Safflower oil
Purslane	Sesame seeds or oil
Salmon	Soybean oil
Sardines	Sunflower oil

LIQUIDS VERSUS SOLIDS

When I look over a picky child's food record, my first question is: Where are the calories coming from—solids or liquids? Babies start out by getting all their calories from fluids, but by nine months they shift to more solid foods. Some babies take their time learning to eat, while others seem to love food from the start.

Typically babies prefer fluids to solids. Many moms encourage their babies to eat more solids by starting meals with solid foods when they are hungriest and less picky. By one year, most kids are getting at least one-quarter of their calories from solid foods. By age three, many kids get roughly half of their calories from solid foods. How many food calories versus liquid calories varies from one child to the next. There is no magic number or ratio.

Yet there are implications for whether calories are coming from solids or liquids. And for any one child it may be better to nudge them toward one or the other.

Situations in which children may need to drink *less*:

- **Children with iron anemia who drink more than thirty-two ounces of milk per day.**
  Too much milk fills them up, and as a result they are less hungry to eat the iron-rich foods they need.

- **Underweight children who drink more than six ounces of juice per day.**
  They don't need more juice. When they drink juice or other sweet drinks throughout the day, it fills them up and they often eat less. I recommend giving water instead.

- **Overweight children who are on the bottle after their first birthday.**
  It's easier and faster to drink through a bottle. Since they don't need extra calories, a cup will slow down the amount they drink and, as a result, reduce calories.

CHECK OUT FLUIDS

Is your child drinking calories instead of munching them?

- Write down everything your child eats or drinks in a "typical" 24-hour day.
- Add up and compare the calories from fluids with those from solid foods. (For calorie counts, read food labels or go online for food composition tables on www.usda.gov.)

When kids drink more than 75 percent of their calories, limiting fluids encourages them to eat more solid foods.

- **Children with a speech delay who are on the bottle after their first birthday.**
  Drinking from a bottle only uses primitive oral-motor movements—as does breast-feeding, but not as much as from a bottle. Using a cup, and eating more solid foods, stimulates the mouth muscles to work harder, which ultimately helps speech. If a child is also underweight, read the next situation.

Situations in which children may need to drink *more*:

- **Underweight children with a speech delay.**
  Sometimes an underweight child with a speech delay needs calories badly enough to justify staying on the bottle longer than is normally recommended. To make the best decision, consult with a pediatric dietitian who can explore all the options for maximizing calories.

- **Children who need extra calories to gain weight.**
  High-calorie, high-nutrient drinks can help kids gain weight. Whether it is a commercial drink or homemade, the best time to drink these is at bedtime. That way they don't interfere with eating meals.

- **Underweight children who drink less than 50 percent of their calories.**
When children don't drink enough calorie-containing fluids, explore why. Although giving high-calorie drinks or trying a new cup are the easiest solutions, they may not be the best. Consider other causes, such as delayed oral-motor skills or sensory problems. Consulting with a speech therapist or a feeding specialist may help.

SLOW DRINKING COULD BE A SIGN OF TROUBLE

If your child *never* drinks 6 ounces in 10 minutes or less, an oral-motor delay could be to blame. Discuss it with your child's pediatrician, especially if growth is a concern.

Filling Nutritional Gaps

If you frequently have a hectic schedule that doesn't leave much time for balanced meals and to handle your kid's quirky food preferences, you may want to be more aggressive in filling in nutritional gaps in your child's eating. There are three main options:

Basic foods
Fortified foods (processed foods that have been enriched with
    vitamins and other nutrients)
Multivitamins

BASIC FOODS
Some foods pack a bigger nutrient punch than others do. Dark leafy vegetables such as spinach, kale, collards, and parsley are loaded with vitamins and minerals. Because these vegetables have

a bitter flavor, most kids won't eat them as is, but will eat them mixed in with other foods. Add chopped parsley to homemade foods such as ground meat, lasagna, or soup. Or try the recipes for Green Veggie Balls and Green Veggie Squares at the end of this chapter.

✕ *Too much of a good thing. Believe it or not, some nutrient-dense foods, when concentrated, can be toxic to infants under three months of age. Home preparation of high-nitrate-containing foods, such as spinach, beets, and carrots, can cause methemoglobinemia, a blood disorder. Don't worry—the risk is minimal in toddlers, older children, and adults.*

Parents who cook can use fruit and vegetable purees to enhance foods. Squash disappears when it is added to soup. Fruit purees and grated carrots disappear in baked foods when they replace part or all of the liquid ingredients.

Many children rely on dairy foods to get enough calcium and protein. When kids don't drink much milk or eat cheese, parents can give concentrated forms of these foods. Powdered milk can be added to pancake or muffin batter. Hard cheeses like Parmesan can be sprinkled on pizza or pasta.

When a child simply doesn't take in enough calories, use the chart below for ideas about foods that can boost calories.

✕ *Do not flavor milk without a reason. Once children taste sweetened, flavored milk, they often refuse to drink plain milk. Use flavored milk only if your child needs extra calories, calcium, or protein.*

To find information about calories or nutrients in foods, try these Web sites: www.calorieking.com, www.nutritiondata.com.

TOO MUCH VITAMIN A . . .

Madison happily ate peaches, cantaloupe, sweet potatoes, spinach, kale, and broccoli from her mother's garden. She also liked such treats from the supermarket as mangoes and apricots. There was only one problem. All of these foods were loaded with vitamin A and, as it turned out, Madison was eating too many, which caused her skin to turn orange.

Dark-green- or orange-colored fruits and vegetables are high in vitamin A. Although there is no health risk from eating too many fruits or vegetables that are high in vitamin A, a common guide is to eat these foods once a day or every other day.

FORTIFIED FOODS

Normally, fresh foods are healthier than processed foods. When foods are processed, naturally occurring nutrients may be lost. Take a vitamin C–containing fruit, such as an orange, and use a heat process to can it. Poof—the vitamin C is destroyed.

Since fresh foods are not always available, processed foods are popular and, at times, more practical. Processed foods are not devoid of nutrients. Over the years, food companies have increasingly enhanced processed foods by adding back what was destroyed, or by adding other nutrients. Technically the terms "enriched" and "fortified" have different meanings. In enriched foods, nutrients lost through processing are restored to the original levels. Fortified foods contain higher levels of nutrients than the food naturally provides. Despite the technical difference, the term "fortified" is generally used whenever vitamins or minerals are added to food.

Fortification has produced clear benefits. For example, the enrichment of grain products began in 1941. Since then nutrition-deficiency diseases, such as beriberi (caused by a lack of thiamine,

FOODS	CALORIES PER SERVING
Avocado	16/tbsp.
Butter/margarine	100/tbsp.
Chocolate syrup	45/tbsp.
Coconut cream	55/tbsp.
Corn syrup	60/tbsp.
Cream, heavy	51/tbsp.
Cream cheese	50/tbsp.
Evaporated milk	25/tbsp.
Flaxseeds	25/tbsp.
Granola	115/oz.
Hummus or bean spreads	17/tbsp.
Jams, jellies, and syrups	52/tbsp.
Milk, powdered (instantized)	15/tbsp.
Mayonnaise	100/tbsp.
Molasses	46/tbsp.
Sour cream	25/tbsp.
Sweetened condensed milk	65/tbsp.
Vegetable oil	110/tbsp.
Wheat germ	25/tbsp.

or vitamin B_1), which was found in the United States at the turn of the century, have become rare.

Although these added nutrients provide benefits, processed foods, even when fortified, tend to be high in sugar, fat, and salt and low in fiber. They are not a nutrition panacea, but they are convenient and popular. Many parents find them useful for filling in nutrition gaps. Kids who can't or won't drink milk can get calcium from orange juice because of fortification.

If you read food labels, you will find that some processed foods offer extra amounts of particular nutrients. Ready-to-eat cereals fall into two groups. One has basic levels of nutrients added, while the second group is superfortified. Since cereals tend to be popular with kids, the superfortified ones can be used for those who need more iron or zinc.

When children older than age one need extra calories and nutrients, special formulas or calorie boosters are often recommended. PediaSure or the lower-costing brands (available at Wal-Mart, Walgreen's, and Target) provide thirty calories per ounce (compared to twenty calories per ounce in whole milk) and all the vitamins and minerals recommended for young children.

Lower in cost and similar in calories are powdered mixes such as Instant Breakfast (made by Nestlé Carnation) and FrescAvena (made by Quaker). When added to whole milk they provide extra vitamins and minerals and boost calories to just over thirty per ounce.

WHAT'S A FORTIFIED FOOD?

A food—usually processed—with extra vitamins or minerals added. Examples include
> Splash and V8 juices
> Calcium-fortified orange juice
> Iron-enriched cereal
> Iodine-fortified salt

MULTIVITAMINS

According to national food surveys, most kids from ages one to five aren't getting the recommended amounts of calcium, vitamin E, and zinc. More than 40 percent aren't getting enough iron.

When children don't eat well, vitamins can be a quick solution to fill in nutrition gaps. But not all children need to take vitamins. Buying vitamins that don't match your child's needs may lead him to take in too much of particular nutrients. Take a closer look at the foods your child eats. Kids who don't drink milk may be getting calcium from fortified foods. Kids who drink fluoridated water don't need extra fluoride.

As a rough guide to which nutrients your child may be missing, look at the nutrients in the food groups your child normally refuses.

Kids who refuse fruits and vegetables may be missing vitamins A and C.
Kids who refuse milk and dairy may be missing calcium, vitamin D, and riboflavin.
Kids who refuse meats may be missing protein, iron, and zinc.
Kids who refuse grains may be missing B vitamins.

The Food and Drug Administration regulates standard vitamins for children under the age of four, ensuring that the nutrient levels are safe. Those for children over the age of four are not regulated and may contain higher levels than is normally recommended.

There are three independent labs that certify the quality of over-the-counter vitamins. You can look for their logos on the labels and learn about warnings and alerts from their Web sites:

U.S. Pharmacopeia (www.usp.org)
Consumer Lab (www.consumerlab.com)
NSF International (www.nsf.org)

If you decide to buy a multivitamin, be warned that there are a dizzying number of choices. How do different brands of vitamins compare? Here's a review of some popular brands.

Poly-Vi-Flor (Mead Johnson)
> Drops for children under age 4
> Chewables for ages 4 to 6

The drops offer nine or more nutrients, and the chewables, ten or more. Different versions are available with and without iron or fluoride. The drops can be mixed with cereal, juice, or fruit. These traditional drops provide reasonable amounts of key nutrients kids may be missing. The different versions enable parents to find the best match for their child's needs. For more details, check the product list at www.meadjohnson.com.

Geber Vitamin Drops
> Drops for ages birth to 3

These provide 100 percent of nine essential nutrients for babies and toddlers. They are a one-size-fits-all version of the more traditional drops available for kids under three. The orange-cherry flavor is more intense than regular vitamin drops and may be more appealing to kids who prefer strong flavors. This is not a good choice for kids who are anemic because it does not contain iron.

Flintstones (Bayer)
> Chewables for 2- and 3-year-olds
> Chewables for 4 years and older

This classic and popular brand of chewable vitamins comes in different formulations. It's available with and without calcium, extra vitamin C, and iron. This may be a good choice for kids with more restricted eating, kids who refuse milk or other calcium-containing foods, or those who don't eat fresh fruits or drink a vitamin C juice every day. Since it provides 100 percent of vitamin A, this is not the best choice for kids who regularly eat orange or deep-colored fruits and vegetables that are naturally high in vitamin A. For more details, check the product list at www.Bayercare.com.

✕ *Kids with asthma need vitamin C. With rising rates of asthma in children, researchers have looked for possible links with diet. One finding is that these kids are often low in vitamin C.*

One A Day Kids Complete
    For ages 4 and up
    ½ tablet for kids 2 to 4
This provides 100 percent of the daily value (DV) for iron, folic acid, and vitamins A, C, D, E, B_6, and B_{12}, and 10 percent of calcium. It has the artificial sweetener aspartame instead of sugar.

✕ *Don't expect to find a full ingredients list on multivitamins. Multivitamins may contain sugar, lactose, and artificial sweeteners, colors, or flavors. If your child has food allergies, look for brands that list ingredients or contact the manufacturer.*

VitaBeans (PharmaLife)
    For ages 4 and up
These chewable jelly beans contain no artificial sweeteners, flavors, or colors. The recommended dose is two jelly beans, which makes it easy to give a lower dose or to give half a dose to a younger child with good chewing skills.

For information on allergy-free vitamins, check out these Web sites: www.nutritionnow.com, www.freedavitamins.com.

Gone are the days of dull, drab multivitamin pills. These days vitamins come in fun shapes—everything from jelly beans, race cars, and action heroes to frozen pops. Kids aren't as likely to reject these fun-looking pills. But don't let the shapes distract you; treat them like medicine.

✕ *Store vitamins out of your child's reach. Even though multivitamins can look more like candy than medicine, they are not. Store them out of your child's reach. Accidental overdose of iron-containing products is the leading cause of fatal poisoning in children under the age of six.*

Recipes

Home-cooked foods can pack in extra nutrition. Try one of these recipes.

✕ Green Veggie Balls

Extra veggies and protein make these a good finger food for toddlers. These freeze well.

2 packages frozen chopped spinach (or other dark, leafy green vegetable), thawed
1 large onion, chopped fine
2 cups herb-flavored stuffing mix
4 eggs
1 stick butter or ½ cup oil
½ tsp. salt
½ tsp. thyme
½ cup grated Parmesan cheese

1. Preheat oven to 350 degrees.
2. Drain spinach to remove as much liquid as possible, then mix with remaining ingredients.
3. Shape into 1-inch balls, then chill for 1 hour.
4. Bake for 15 minutes.

✕ Green Veggie Squares

This recipe is high in calories, protein, and fiber. It can be frozen and reheated.

4 tbsp. butter or margarine
2 packages frozen chopped spinach or other green leafy vegetable, thawed and well-drained, or 2 pounds fresh, cooked and drained
3 eggs
1 tsp. salt
1 pound Cheddar cheese, grated
1 tbsp. finely minced onion
1 cup flour (Optional: substitute 2 tbsp. of the flour with wheat germ)
1 cup milk
1 tsp. baking powder

1. Preheat oven to 350 degrees.
2. Melt butter or margarine in a 9-by-13-inch pan.
3. In a large bowl, mix together the spinach with all the remaining ingredients. Pour into pan.
4. Bake for 35 minutes.
5. Cool, then cut into 1-inch squares.

✗ Yogurt-Fruit Smoothie

Use frozen fruits to make this a cool, icy drink.

1 cup yogurt
1 banana
½ cup fruit (any combination of fresh, frozen, or canned)
Optional: 3 tbsp. powdered milk

Mix in a blender until smooth.

✗ Breakfast Drink 1

For kids who don't eat much at breakfast, try this high-calorie drink (44 calories per ounce).

1 cup whole milk
½ cup dry baby cereal
½ cup fruit (fresh, canned, or frozen)
2 tsp. vegetable oil

Mix all ingredients together in a blender until smooth.

✗ Breakfast Drink 2

This drink made with peanut butter is similar to the one above and slightly higher in calories (50 calories per ounce).

1 cup whole milk
1 package Carnation Instant Breakfast

2 tbsp. peanut butter
½ cup fruit
¼ cup dry baby cereal

Mix all ingredients together in a blender until smooth.

✕ Bean Milk Shake

When I offered this shake to a support group of parents with picky eaters, I had few takers. Nonetheless, I know families and kids who like it. This unusual recipe is high in calories, protein, and fiber, and tastes better than it sounds.

½ pound dry pinto beans (or a 16-oz. can of any white mild-flavored bean)
1 can sweetened condensed milk
1 tsp. vanilla
1 tsp. cinnamon
½ tsp. nutmeg

1. Rinse the beans and put them in saucepan. (If using canned beans, rinse thoroughly and skip to step 3.) Add 3 cups of water and bring to a boil. Let sit for 1 hour.

2. Rinse and add new water, then simmer for 1 hour or until soft.

3. Put the beans into a blender. Add 1½ cups of water and remaining ingredients. Process until smooth and creamy. Refrigerate overnight.

✕ Apple Carrot Squares

Use these not-too-sweet squares as a substitute for muffins.

1 cup flour
1 tsp. baking soda
½ tsp. cinnamon
¼ cup vegetable oil
½ cup brown sugar
1 egg
⅔ cup applesauce
⅓ cup grated carrots
Optional: ½ cup chopped walnuts, 1 tbsp. wheat germ

1. Preheat oven to 350 degrees.
2. Mix together the flour and baking soda. Set aside.
3. Mix all the remaining ingredients, then add the flour mixture.
4. Pour into a greased 7-inch square pan.
5. Bake for 45 minutes.

✕ Pumpkin Raisin Squares

These easy-to-freeze squares provide extra vitamin A. Use them for snacks or dessert.

¼ cup vegetable oil
¾ cup brown sugar
⅔ cup pumpkin puree (not *pie filling*)
2 eggs
⅔ cup flour

¾ tsp. cinnamon
½ tsp. ground ginger
¾ tsp. baking powder
¼ tsp. baking soda
½ cup raisins
Optional: ½ cup chopped nuts, 1 tbsp. wheat germ

1. Preheat oven to 350 degrees.
2. Beat together the vegetable oil, sugar, pumpkin, and eggs.
3. Mix the flour with remaining dry ingredients and add to liquid mix.
4. Pour into a greased 9-inch square pan.
5. Bake for 30 minutes.

You'll find more recipes and ideas in these books:

- *The Mom's Guide to Meal Makeovers* by Janice Bissex and Liz Weiss
- *Secrets to Feeding a Healthy Family* by Ellen Satter

As a parent who cares about helping your child develop a healthy attitude toward food, you'll need to be flexible about the foods your child eats. At times, this means letting your child eat too much of one food and not enough of another. Good nutrition is important for maximizing health, but children need to learn this on their own.

Do
- Limit the junk foods you have in your house. They are not good for you, either.
- Check whether your child is drinking fluoridated water.

- Try omega-3 enriched eggs or other foods high in this essential fatty acid.
- Use multivitamins if your child is not regularly eating foods from the four basic food groups.
- If growth is an issue, boost calories with supplements of high calorie foods.

DON'T
- Allow your child to fill up on liquids. Encourage a balance between solids and liquids.
- Use flavored milk unless your child needs the extra calories, protein, or calcium.
- Restrict your child's fat intake without a reason. Normally young children need more fat than adults do.
- Use an iron-containing multivitamin unless your child is anemic or at risk for anemia.

Making Food Desirable

Before kids open their mouths for food, they look at it, and sometimes, even without tasting it, decide not to eat it. This tendency has frustrated parents for generations. To circumvent picky-eater food refusals, parents try various inducements. And some of them work, some of the time.

This chapter takes a deeper look at the strategies that parents and professionals use to entice picky eaters into eating. It also describes design features in cups and utensils that can make eating easier and offers a list of food picture books that may inspire food discussions with your child.

Playful Enticements

Do preschoolers eat better when food looks "cute"? Does tuna salad look more appealing when it's shaped into a porcupine with pretzel quills? According to a Colorado State University study on preschool snacks, it doesn't matter. Serving three- to five-year-old children snacks like bagel baseballs and muffin faces rather than the same foods in a regular form didn't sway them. They ate equal amounts of food regardless of whether it was dressed up or not. The results surprise those who have watched picky eaters eat "ants on a log" (raisins, peanut butter, and celery), smiley-faced apples, and other fanciful foods. Why didn't the cute foods in the Colorado State University study entice preschoolers to eat more?

It may be because there was no emphasis on the social context. When researchers have studied the effects of social environment on food choices, they have found that it matters. Several studies have demonstrated that family and peers influence which foods children eat or don't eat.

This is not surprising if one considers the basic fact that children learn by watching. So if parents can influence a child's food choices, how should they go about doing it? Beyond being a good role model, the answer is to do it on the child's level and keep the focus on the food.

One mother encourages her two-year-old daughter to eat broccoli by emphasizing the tree shape and asking her if she wants to eat the leaves or the trunk. With each bite her daughter chooses which part she wants, and soon she has eaten the entire broccoli stalk. Three-year-old Brandon is learning to count, and his father makes a game of eating more food by counting the bites. A grandmother proudly told me how she entices her grandchildren to eat spinach with "food magic." She takes a pot full of spinach, covers it, and puts it over the burner. She waves her hands and, *abracadabra,* when she lifts the lid, the spinach has shrunk. Watching bread rise or muffins bake are other examples of "food magic."

With imagination, there's no end to the whimsy you can add to food. Just remember that for a child who is easily overwhelmed or uncomfortable with new foods, it's better to go slowly. If a child feels pressured to eat, no matter how well-intentioned or playfully presented, it will still not be fun.

Rachel, a former teacher, kept a watchful eye on what Eric, her eighteen-month-old son, ate. She knew that Eric hadn't eaten meat in three days and was worried about his protein intake. So she decided to make a big deal out of the chicken she was roasting for dinner. She not only made sure to talk about it, she encouraged her son to smell it and watch it cook. To heighten the suspense, several times when they peered into the oven, she asked aloud, "I wonder if it is ready?"

Sure enough, Eric tuned in to the message his mother was sending. Something special was happening. He went along with the magical mood, and so Rachel's efforts paid off. That night, Eric ate chicken.

If you watch your child closely, you can invent other simple games that are fun and effective. But in order to work, games need to match a child's interests and learning style. Even then, they may not work, and, as with all games, it's important to be a good sport. If a child doesn't go along with the game, don't act disappointed, upset, or angry. Children eat best when they feel like it is their idea.

BE PLAYFUL, RATHER THAN SNEAKY

Be aware that in some instances, well-intentioned parents feel they are being playful with food, yet their children experience it differently. A typical scenario is when a child refuses food, and her parents look for ways to circumvent the veto, normally by hiding or camouflaging the vegetables and other foods that the child rejected.

Making objectionable food less visible can take different forms. One mother grates veggies into omelettes or tomato sauce; another uses a sandwich press to encase vegetables and cheese; one father rolls up everything in a tortilla.

Of course, there's nothing inherently wrong with adding extra ingredients to enhance the food your child eats. But it is not something to be done carelessly. You don't want your child to become suspicious of the food you offer. If your child feels he has been tricked into eating something he doesn't want, he's likely to be resentful and become wary of all food you encourage. In the long run, being sneaky with your child's food can create more problems than it solves.

Your child is less likely to react negatively if you add ingredients that make foods healthier for everyone in the family. Add grated carrots to sauce, or flaxseed meal or wheat germ to pancake batter. Make zucchini bread or buy foods that are nutrient-dense. Try cereal bars, hummus, bean spreads, fortified cereals, and juices.

Food Presentation and Cooking

Pointing out food's flavors, colors, and shapes helps children to focus on food. On a practical level, the size, shape, and texture of food can also make it easier for a young child to hold or eat it.

While Megan was at work, her husband reheated sixteen-month-old Caleb's favorite dinner: meat loaf, potatoes, and peas. But Caleb didn't eat. When Megan came home and saw the dish on the counter, she knew why. All the food was lumped together in one big bowl. Megan normally paid attention to food details such as:

- **Size of the pieces**
  Caleb, like many toddlers, preferred to eat with his hands rather than a spoon. Megan normally cut his food into small pieces so that it was easier for him to pick up.

- **Amount**
  Instead of filling a bowl with food, Megan gave him a few pieces at a time. Not only did Caleb eat more this way, it also stopped him from overstuffing his mouth.

- **Texture**
  Caleb could be surprisingly fussy. If the peas were the wrong brand and just a little tougher to chew, he didn't eat them.

✕ *Children with rigid resistance to new foods need special handling. By providing more structure and a gradual food progression, extremely fussy children learn to eat new foods. For more details on this read chapter 12, "Feeding a Child with Special Needs."*

COOKING

Home cooking also helps to entice children to eat. There's the aroma of food, and the opportunity to watch the preparation, which can be an exciting event for kids.

Flavor Counts

When cooking for kids, a common mistake parents make is to assume that food needs to be bland. However, many parents tell me their children eat better when they stop using baby food and serve more flavorful table food. Of course, the optimal degree of flavor intensity will vary from one child to another. In countries where spicy foods are popular, after age two children are gradually introduced to spicier foods. By age four or five, most of these children have learned to enjoy the burn of hot, spicy foods.

Herbs do more than add flavor; many have medicinal properties and need to be used with care when given to young children. According to a respected reference on the safety of herbs, the following are not recommended for young children: aloe, fennel oil, horseradish, mint oil, nasturtium, peppermint oil, senna leaf and pod, and watercress.

In terms of increasing food appeal, it has long been known that toddlers like salt. More than twenty years ago, researchers reported that two-year-olds ate more soup and other foods with higher amounts of salt. By age four, salty pretzels were more popular than the plain ones.

Because home-cooked foods do not need as much salt as processed foods to convey the same level of saltiness, home cooking cuts down the amount of salt your child eats. Compared to more processed foods, almost anything you cook at home, using basic ingredients, will be lower in salt. Compare the sodium in the following foods:

1 cup quick or old-fashioned oatmeal (3 mg) versus 1 package instant flavored oatmeal (260 mg)

½ cup frozen vegetables (48 mg) versus ½ cup frozen vegetables with flavored sauce (400 mg)

4 oz. chicken breast (without skin), roasted (36 mg) versus ½ package chicken entrée with sauce (338 mg)

You don't have to get rid of salt totally. The human body needs salt. Young children from two to five years of age need at least 300 milligrams of sodium per day. There are 600 milligrams of sodium in 1/4 teaspoon salt. The justification to reduce salt is based on the fact that Americans consume an excessive amount, which, later in life, is linked to hypertension.

Be Sensitive to a Child's Changing Needs

Ease children into eating adult fare by considering both a child's ability to bite and chew and her ability to self-feed with a spoon or fork. Easy-to-chew foods such as pasta, rice, mashed potatoes, and squash are popular when babies sit and wait to be fed, and again later, after they learn to feed themselves with utensils. In between, it is good to include at least one finger food at each meal.

For toddlers who want finger foods but aren't quite ready for grilled-cheese sandwiches, try toasted pocket sandwiches. Toast a single slice of bread. Cut it in half, then take a dull knife and gently insert it along the cut edge, prying the toasted sides apart to form a pocket. Fill it with cheese, sliced meat, or another filling.

For older toddlers and preschoolers who are eating raw fruits and vegetables, you can make them softer by zapping them briefly in a microwave oven. Or you can make them more fun and substantial by adding a dip, such as hummus, plain yogurt mixed with salad dressing or seasoned with dill and lemon juice or some other spice mix, or tahini mixed with water and lemon juice.

Cooking Activities

As kids grow older, most are eager to help in the kitchen. And generally, the more involved kids are with food, the more likely they will eat it.

For parents ready to take on the challenge, first be sure to protect an overeager child from the hazards of knives, hot surfaces, and electrical appliances.

When it's time to cook, kids can stir, knead, roll, pour, and dump ingredients into a bowl. You can also try some of the following:

Gadgets

Old-fashioned, hand-powered gadgets such as apple-peeling machines, orange squeezers, ice-cream makers, egg beaters, and even potato mashers fascinate preschoolers. Turning cranks and manipulating beaters is fun. As the project proceeds, talk about the oranges or other food being prepared, so they'll be excited about trying the final product.

Shakes

Simple shakes can be mixed in a jar, which a child helps to "shake." When kids need to drink more milk, here are some simple ones. Try mixing and shaking

Equal amounts of milk and yogurt (without fruit chunks)
Fruit juice with a jar of baby fruit
Milk with a spoonful of instant-pudding mix

Popsicle Sticks

Allow your child to spear Popsicle sticks into banana chunks, melon cubes, and other soft foods. This also makes them easier to hold and more fun to eat.

Sandwiches

For simple sandwich roll-ups, let kids flatten bread with a rolling pin, then spread with a filling and roll it up.

Shakers

Buy small shakers and fill them with wheat germ or grated cheese. Kids love the opportunity to use a shaker and will want to shake it onto their own food. If they want to go overboard, you'll need to limit the amount, which may even increase the appeal.

Spreads

Young children can safely spread their favorite goop onto bread or crackers with a plastic knife. Spreadables include the dips mentioned on page 127 or cottage cheese mixed with fruit or tuna. For children past the age of allergy risk, there's a high-calorie peanut spread you can make by mixing equal amounts of peanut butter and butter and sweetening it with honey. For kids who can't eat peanut butter or other nuts, soy spreads are available in health-food stores.

Eating Gear

There are a dizzying number of cups, plates, and spoons to choose from. Which one should you buy? Does your child need a sippy cup or will an open cup do?

Most parents end up with a cabinet full of cups and other eating paraphernalia. They discover that as a child moves through different stages, some work better than others, at least for a while.

Normally, you won't need to make changes unless your child is having a problem taking in enough calories. Ryan was taken off the bottle at eighteen months. I saw him three months later because his growth rate had dropped. Because his fluids were low, changing his cup to one that was easier for him to drink from helped him to get the extra calories he needed. Emma was a busy bee who always squirmed to leave the table. Giving her a bowl and big-girl utensils helped her to sit at the table longer.

When a child is stuck or in need of extra help, fine-tuning eating gear can

- Increase the fun factor
- Make it easier to take in more food
- Make it easier to self-feed

Changing your child's eating equipment can be a simple solution to a potentially complex problem. The following list of products includes those used by specialists to help children with specific feeding problems. If your child needs extra help with eating or self-feeding, the trial-and-error approach takes time. For some children, this makes eating overly frustrating. Consult with a feeding specialist to shorten the process, as the trained eye of a specialist can recognize problems that parents sometimes miss.

CUPS

Most parents go through a trial-and-error phase with a baby's first cup. With practice, babies eventually learn to drink from a cup. But before weaning your child off the bottle or breast, she needs to drink well enough from the cup to meet her fluid and calorie needs. Typically, this means being able to drink four ounces within ten minutes.

Generally, older babies use short, two-handled cups (which are easier to hold) with soft spouts (which are easier to drink from). Toddlers typically use more rugged cups with or without handles and with hard, spill-proof spouts. Preschoolers may opt for the straw tops or the snazzy sports-type bottles.

Cup Drinking 101

To make early cup drinking easier, give your child some practice with an open cup. To control the flow, adjust the tilt of the cup as you hold it to your child's lips. Then follow these tips:

- Offer a thickened liquid. This moves slowly, and gives a child more time to coordinate the movements of the jaw, lips, and tongue. Depending on a child's age and calorie needs, it could be:

    formula or breast milk mixed with cereal
    fruit puree diluted with juice
    yogurt and milk
    a fruit shake or smoothie

tex is available at Wal-Mart, Target, and Kmart. When a child's lips press against the inner seal, the liquid flows out. *Infa-Trainer* is available from New Visions. With this cup, the lid allows you to adjust the flow rate by turning the top.

Training Systems

Several companies make training systems that provide a cup with a variety of tops. These usually include a nipple, straw, and spout. They can make the transition from bottle to cup easier. They are also good for kids who learn to drink from a straw before they learn how to hold a cup.

Insulated Cups

These keep drinks cold, making it safer to take milk in a cup for short trips without an ice pack. Gerber and The First Years make these.

Sip-Tip Cup

This specialty cup makes it easier to learn how to drink through a straw. It has a one-way valve, which keeps the liquid in the straw. A lid holds the straw in place and, when pressed, pushes liquid up the straw. All the parts and an additional mouthpiece are sold separately from New Visions.

Weighted Cups

These are harder to tip over and help kids who need more sensory input.

Baby Cup Feeder

This tiny cup holds 1.5 ounces. It is sometimes recommended by specialists for babies who do not take enough fluid from the bottle or breast. It's available from Beyond Play.

SPOONS

There's an endless variety of spoons to choose from. Temperature-sensitive spoons let you know that food is too hot. Some spoons stand upright to avoid contact with germy surfaces. While these are potentially useful features, they don't help children to eat more or to self-feed. To do that, you need to consider other, not-quite-so-obvious design features.

Material

First and foremost, a spoon needs to be sturdy enough to withstand rough handling, namely, unpredictable amounts of banging, biting, or dropping. For this reason, picnic-type disposable spoons are too flimsy and can be unsafe. These are different than the newer disposables that are sturdy enough to be reused, yet affordable.

Rubber-coated or hard plastic spoons feel more gentle in the mouth than a metal spoon, especially when teeth are coming in or gums are sensitive. Many children bite metal spoons. One way to discourage this is to use plastic.

Bowl Size and Shape

The part of the spoon that enters the mouth—the bowl—should be sized in proportion to a child's mouth. The shape—its depth or shallowness—affects the amount of work needed to remove the food. A deep bowl requires more work. The upper lip needs to move farther downward to scrape food off the spoon completely.

Handle Size and Shape

Handles can be long or short, fat or skinny, straight or curved. Long handles are useful early on; they provide the extra room that's needed when a child needs adult help to guide the spoon. Later, short handles or ones with a loop shape are easier for small

hands to grab. Thick, fat handles are easier for small hands to hold. Curved handles can help food reach the mouth when a child has not learned how to flex the wrist.

Spoon Design Considerations
- Instead of a solid bowl, you can find ones with a perforated surface, which traps food. This design makes it easier for food to stick to the spoon.
- A safety shield between the handle and the bowl prevents a child from putting the spoon too far back in the mouth.
- Spoons can stand upright on a suction base. This is intended to limit contact with dirty surfaces and avoid germs.
- Bowl surfaces are normally smooth, but are available with a textured bottom surface. This can be helpful for children with oral-sensory needs.
- Temperature-sensitive spoons indicate when food is too hot.
- Bright colors, patterns, or cartoon or superhero characters all increase the fun factor.

SPECIALIZED SPOONS
Maroon Spoon
Because of its flat bowl, this hard plastic spoon is a favorite among feeding specialists. It comes in two sizes.

Textured Spoon
This spoon is designed for children who are making the transition to spoon-feeding as part of an oral-stimulation program.

Steady Spoon
This easy-to-hold spoon helps children with poor coordination who are three years and older. It keeps food balanced on the spoon until it gets to the mouth. For more information, call, toll-free, 877-849-2273, or look online at www.handlecare.com.

FORKS

Using a fork requires a more precise and focused action: aiming for a specific piece of food. You can help your child with this by offering foods that are easy to stab: cut-up chunks of potato, banana, grilled cheese, or other firm foods. Later, offer soft, slippery, or crumbly foods such as noodles or pancakes.

Most of the same design features that affect spoon handles apply to forks. But there are a few differences. Does your child need a fork with blunt or pointed tines? The blunt edges are a safety feature. Because parents are less likely to guide a fork, it's best to pick a fork with a short handle. The closer a child's hand is to the prong end, the easier it will be to use.

DISHES

Before children start to self-feed, they enjoy seeing a character on the bottom of the bowl that emerges when the food covering it is eaten.

Once kids begin to self-feed, practical considerations become more important.

- Bowls with a raised ridge make it easier to scoop food onto a spoon. Flat plates are better later, when spearing food with a fork.
- Suction bottoms help bowls stay put and not topple over.

Special training plates and scooper bowls are available from Beyond Play.

Almost all cups, bowls, and dishes are made of plastic, unless you find or inherit an old set. Even the newer disposables for children are sturdy enough to reuse. But don't ever use Styrofoam. Kids sometimes bite these, which is dangerous.

OTHER GEAR

Baby Safe Feeder

Food is tucked inside a mesh bag. As a child bites down, the food is effectively pureed as it passes through the mesh. This allows a child who wants to bite but whose chewing skills are inconsistent to try new food textures while avoiding the risk of choking. The mesh top is washable and reusable and screws onto a base with an easy-to-hold handle. This is available at Beyond Play, New Visions, Babies "R" Us, and a variety of retail stores.

Whistling Straws

These are both fun and practical. They assist in self-feeding and various oral skills. They are available at New Visions.

High Chair Helper

This is a special insert that slides into a high chair to help a young child sit upright. It is available at Babies "R" Us.

Nonskid Mats

When placed on the seat of a high chair, these can prevent a child from sliding forward. When placed under a bowl, they keep it in place, making it easier to scoop a spoon against it. Look for perforated plastic mats that can be cut up or buy products designed for this from specialty sources such as Beyond Play.

SOURCES

If you don't find the items you want in local stores, try these other sources:

Specialty Stores
Beyond Play
1442A Walnut St. #52

Berkeley, CA 94709
877-428-1244 (toll-free)
www.beyondplay.com

The Equipment Shop
P.O. Box 33
Bedford, MA 01730
800-525-7681
www.equipmentshop.com

New Visions
1124 Roberts Mountain Rd.
Faber, VA 22938
804-361-2285
www.new-vis.com

Web Sites
www.babyant.com
www.babysupermall.com
www.greatbabyproducts.com
www.babyuniverse.com
www.gerber.com
www.playtex.com
www.thefirstyears.com

Reading About Food

A story can spark curiosity and inspire a child to adopt a new attitude or try a new food, if not today, then tomorrow. Look for books that send positive food messages, stimulate curiosity, and help expand your child's food vocabulary.

Here's a partial list of books that make food fun:

Alligator Arrived with Apples: A Potluck Alphabet Feast by Crescent Dragonwagon. Alladin, 1992.

An alphabet book that expands a child's vocabulary for naming vegetarian foods.

Anansi and the Talking Melon by Eric Kimmel. Holiday House, 1995.

A story about a spider who overeats melon.

The Beastly Feast by Bruce Goldstone. Henry Holt, 1998.

Animals come together to have a feast that includes peas and rice.

Blueberries for Sal by Robert McClosky. Puffin, 1976.

An adventurous tale about picking blueberries.

Bread, Bread, Bread by Ann Morris. HarperTrophy, 1993.

Explores the many forms of bread throughout the world.

Bread and Jam for Frances by Russell Hoban. HarperCollins, 1964.

In this classic story, a little badger discovers that eating the same foods day after day is not much fun.

Bread Is for Eating by David and Phillis Gershator. Henry Holt, 1995.

A story that answers an obvious question.

The Carrot Seed by Ruth Kraus. Harper, 1945.

An inspiring story about a boy's steadfast belief and care in planting a carrot seed.

Chicken Soup with Rice: A Book of Months by Maurice Sendak. HarperCollins, 1962.

Describes the pleasures of each month and how each season is nice, when eating a bowl of chicken soup with rice.

D.W. the Picky Eater by Marc Brown. Little Brown, 1997.

A story about a picky eater who finds numerous foods disgusting but eventually eats and learns a lesson.

Eating Fractions by Bruce McMillan. Scholastic, 1991.

A book that cleverly combines math and food. It includes recipes and suggestions for using math skills for measuring ingredients.

Eating the Alphabet: Fruits and Vegetables from A to Z by Lois Ehlert. Red Wagon Books, 1996.
This board book introduces children to a colorful variety of fruits and vegetables.

Green Eggs and Ham by Dr. Seuss. Random House, 1960.
This classic story teaches that adventurous eating is worth a try.

Gregory the Terrible Eater by Mitchell Sharmat. Four Winds, 1980.
A goat rejects the usual goat fare in favor of fruits, vegetables, eggs, and orange juice.

Growing Vegetable Soup by Lois Ehlert. Voyager Books, 1990.
Describes the details about a vegetable garden that provides the ingredients to make the best vegetable soup. It includes a recipe.

I Will Never, Not Ever, Eat a Tomato by Lauren Child. Candlewick Press, 2000.
An endearing story about Lola, a fussy eater, that illustrates how food dislikes are often based on preconceptions rather than taste buds.

Lunch by Denise Fleming. Henry Holt, 1998.
In this board book, a hungry mouse nibbles his way through a vegetarian feast.

Mufaro's Beautiful Daughters by John Steptoe. Lothrop, 1987.
In this African tale, yams and sunflower seeds are given and received as well-appreciated gifts.

Oliver's Fruit Salad by Vivian French. Orchard Books, 1998.
Oliver helps his grandfather grow and pick fruits, yet he refuses to eat them. At last, his grandfather makes a bountiful fruit salad that Oliver eats and eats.

Oliver's Vegetables by Vivian French. Orchard Books, 1998.
Oliver learns to like vegetables with his grandfather's help.

One Hundred Hungry Ants by Elinor J. Pinczes. Houghton Mifflin (reprint), 1999.
A whimsical tale that introduces math by recounting how ants march off for a picnic.

Pancakes, Pancakes! by Eric Carle. Knopf, 1970.
Cornflakes won't do for a determined lad who insists on his favorite breakfast and who is required to gather all the needed ingredients.

Pumpkin, Pumpkin by Jeanne Titherington. HarperTrophy, 1990.
A beautifully illustrated book about growing pumpkins.

Stone Soup by Ann McGovern. Scholastic, 1986.
A clever traveler tricks an old woman into making a hearty soup.

Vegetable Soup: The Nutritional ABC's and *The Fruit Bowl: A Contest Among the Fruit* (two books in one) by Dianne Warren and Susan Smith Jones. Oasis Publications, 1996.

The Very Hungry Caterpillar by Eric Carle. Putnam Publishing Group, 1984.
This popular book teaches counting and the days of the week while describing a caterpillar eating through an apple, a pear, plums, cherry pie, and sausage.

Yoko and Friends by Rosemary Wells. Hyperion, 1998.
In this board book a mother asks, "What would you like for lunch today?" The answer turns out to be sushi.

For a more comprehensive list of young children's books about food, read *Pot Luck: A Feast of Picture Books About Food* by Kimberly Hoblet.

Depending on your family and your child's personality, making food desirable can take many forms. Whether it's reading a book, cooking, or trying a new cup, your child's reaction will guide you as to what works and what doesn't.

Do
- Make food feel like an adventure rather than a chore.
- Experiment with presentation.
- Allow your child to help in the kitchen.
- Make eating easier by offering more finger foods.
- Look at the design of cups and utensils if your child needs help with self-feeding.
- Talk or read about food.

Don't
- Act upset when your child doesn't appreciate the food you offer.
- Expect that making food cute will improve your child's eating.
- Give your child a reason to be wary about food. If you need to add extra ingredients, do it with care.

Food Textures and Flavors

I s there any rhyme or reason behind a picky eater's food refusals? Not all food refusals are arbitrary. Although they can seem to come out of the blue, sometimes a child's decision to refuse or accept a food is linked to the food's texture or flavor. Two-year-old Andy eats only chicken nuggets, Cheerios, crackers, and French fries—all crunchy, a favorite texture among toddlers.

Looking for patterns in food refusals is a useful strategy when children need to overcome sensory integration dysfunction or motor delays, which make eating a struggle. There is an inherent difference between a child who *does not want* to eat and one who is *uncomfortable* or *unable* to eat.

Kids can be amazingly fussy—to the point of eating only one brand of chicken nuggets. Or they may eat pasta, but only without sauce. Sometimes kids with rigid food preferences have underlying sensory or motor issues, which if addressed will improve eating. And sometimes rigid food preferences are really not about food at all, but are about control, which is related to developmental needs.

Patterns of Food Refusal

FOOD JAGS

Does your child eat a food for weeks on end and then suddenly, without any apparent reason, refuse to eat it? Then, a few weeks later, accept that food again? Erratic food preferences are a norm among toddlers. Although hard to live with, often the best reaction is to ignore it.

In some children food jags follow a different pattern. Instead of fluctuating food likes and dislikes, there's a downward spiral in the number of acceptable foods. If your child's food jags continue for months rather than weeks, with favorite foods dropped and never regained as acceptable, with an end result of an ever more restrictive list of acceptable foods (though the exact number is debatable, I use six as a guide), then you'll want to take them more seriously.

Avoid giving your child *exactly* the same foods every day. Rotate the food your child eats over three days and gradually expand the variety by using the flavor-to-flavor or texture-to-texture strategies described later in this chapter. You'll find other suggestions on rigid food preferences in chapter 12, "Feeding a Child with Special Needs."

APPETITE FLUCTUATIONS

Does your child eat everything one day and nothing the next? This is another common toddler behavior. Ignoring it helps kids outgrow this stage faster. Continue to offer regular meals and snacks. Don't get angry, but don't offer endless substitute choices, both of which encourage food refusal.

TEXTURE PREFERENCES

Does your child eat only dry, crunchy foods? This preference is common in young children. These foods are familiar, easy to pick up, and easy to eat. But for some children there's more to it. If your child is stuck on a particular food texture, you'll need to determine whether or not it is simply a passing phase.

When the texture preference is related to immature oral skills or sensory issues, waiting can make these issues worse. Struggles over food make eating stressful and unpleasant for parents and children. If your child has any of the following, seek help:

- **Vomiting or choking**
  If choking or vomiting is a regular occurrence and there's no medical explanation, hypersensitivity to texture may be the cause. Mouthing toys help to desensitize the mouth. Kids who never go through a mouthing phase are more likely to react to food texture and benefit from therapy.

- **Refusal to eat foods that require chewing**
  Does your child refuse to eat foods that require chewing? Toddlers with short attention spans may not want to take the time to sit and eat. Or a child with immature feeding skills may not be ready to eat more difficult foods.

- **Problems eating lumpy or mixed-texture foods**
  Does your child reject lumpy foods? These are more difficult to eat and can be frightening for a child with immature eating skills. Try increasing textures gradually and avoiding foods that combine purees or liquids with chunkier solids.

- **Refusing to be spoon-fed**
  This is both common and normal in young children as they are struggling to gain independence. Often toddlers refuse to eat food from a spoon, not because of texture but because they prefer to feed themselves. Even if given a spoon to eat

on their own, they may reject it because it's more work or awkward to use. At this stage many prefer finger foods.

✕ *Read the chart about food texture progression (see page 150) to make eating easier. Most kids under the age of three have immature feeding skills. When kids have problems related to food texture, a simple solution is to give foods that are easier to eat and gradually introduce those that are more difficult.*

FLAVOR PREFERENCES

For years, candy makers and feeding therapists have used the appeal of tart or sour flavors to entice kids. Now there's research to justify it. Formal studies by Julie Mennella, a biopsychologist from the Monell Institute, demonstrated that five-year-olds enjoy the taste of concentrated citric acid.

Why do some kids eat better when food is bland, salty, sweet, or spicy? The answer is partly genetic and partly conditioning. Academics offer theories that explain flavor preferences related to a child's age and history. There's a great deal of evidence demonstrating that early food experiences predispose babies to enjoy a greater variety of food flavors. (For more on this, see the last section in chapter 4, "Fussy Babies.") On a practical level, it seems that babies tend to prefer sweet tastes, toddlers salty, and older preschoolers tart.

RIGID PREFERENCES FOR DULL FOOD COLORS

Kids tend to like bright colors in toys, balloons, clothes, and even furniture. Yet when it comes to food, a surprising number prefer the dullest colors: white, beige, and brown. Where does this come from?

One theory is that a dull color preference really isn't about color at all but more likely about flavor and familiarity. Scientists speculate that biologically it makes sense for young children to prefer familiar foods—out in nature, these would be the least likely to be poisonous.

In the first comprehensive survey of adult picky eaters, Dr. Jane Kauer, an anthropologist from the University of Pennsylvania, found a "master list" of foods that are universally accepted: fried chicken, French fries, chocolate chip cookies, and Kraft macaroni and cheese. Sound familiar? If you substitute chicken nuggets for fried chicken, this could be a "master list" for toddler picky eaters.

Another theory associates rigid food preferences with social development. Based on her survey with adult picky eaters, Dr. Kauer found that the fussiest eaters had lost touch with the social context of food. For adult picky eaters, the strongest motivator to eat a food they hated was social context. The majority admitted they would eat something they hated rather than offend a host. Only the fussiest of the adult picky eaters were unfazed by the social ramifications of refusing food. This is an interesting observation. Those who work with autistic kids recognize the pattern for both rigid food habits and struggles with social interactions.

✕ *Kids with rigid food preferences that are typical in autism need special handling. Kids with autism or a related diagnosis often have rigid food preferences based on color, flavor, texture, or temperature. As the number of these kids grows, professionals are gaining insights into what works. (For details on this, see the section on rigid food preferences in chapter 12, "Feeding a Child with Special Needs.")*

Sensory Dimensions of Food

When kids reject food, the first thing we tend to think is that they don't like the taste. From my experience, often the problem is texture. Texture, the tactile dimension of food when it enters the mouth, is important because it determines how hard or easy a food is to eat, and because some children are surprisingly sensitive to it.

The feel of food in your mouth can add to the pleasure of eating. After months of mush, imagine the new sensations evoked by a Cheerio, or the fun of hearing a crunch from biting into a cracker. But tactile and sensory food experiences are not always fun, especially early on. For babies and young children, foods with interesting textures present challenges. They require new skills and new ways of moving and coordinating the muscles in the mouth. Kids are not always ready for the challenge.

At nine months, Kyle began to vomit regularly. Because of a strong family history of food allergies, his mother assumed it was an allergic reaction. Months later, after a work-up with an allergist, an elimination diet, and a serious drop-off in growth, it turned out that Kyle did not have food allergies. He vomited because he was highly sensitive to mixed food textures.

Kyle had done well with smooth baby foods. The trouble started later, with the transition to table foods. It was the stage three foods that threw him off—somehow, the combination of mush and small bits of food didn't work. Whenever he ate these foods, Kyle threw up. At the time, everyone focused on his risk for allergies and, as a result, missed the real problem.

Kyle was so sensitive to food texture that it interfered with his growth and his ability to eat table foods. With the help of a therapist and a nutritionist he overcame his problems. The therapist used a vibrator, at first on Kyle's face and later in his mouth to reduce his sensitivity. The nutritionist suggested changes in Kyle's formula (to increase calories and reduce the risk for an allergic reaction). She also helped Kyle's mother increase textures gradually, at first by using thickeners and later by giving Kyle crunch-and-crumble foods that dissolve quickly (see the chart on page 150). With these changes Kyle's vomiting decreased and he slowly began eating more table foods.

Not all food sensitivities cause eating problems. In fact, mild sensitivities are likely to go unnoticed. One mother, remembering her son, Rafael, as a baby, said, "Oh, he loved his milk. He drank nothing else, no water, no juice, nothing but milk." I asked if she thickened his milk (or, more accurately, formula), perhaps with cereal. "Oh, yes," she answered. In her native Colombia, cereal was routinely added to a baby's milk.

Even without added cereal, milk is thicker than water. For a child with emerging skills, that difference, though subtle, makes swallowing easier. Thicker liquids have more body, move more slowly, and, as a result, provide more sensations. All this helps to coordinate the movements needed to swallow.

Commercial thickeners are routinely added to liquids when adults have swallowing problems (usually after suffering a stroke). Unless there is a recognized problem with swallowing or growth, these thickeners are not recommended for babies drinking from a bottle. Babies tend to adapt and the goal is to encourage development of the needed skills rather than to make things easier. For more on thickeners, see page 156.

✕ *Use a shake to make learning how to drink from a cup easier. Make those first sips from a cup (preferably an open one) easier. Use a shake or other thick drink and gently support the chin to keep the lower lip in contact with the cup. This helps kids learn how to drink from a cup with fewer drools or spills. You don't need to do this every time, or for very long. Most kids learn fast, but this speeds up the process.*

The move from liquids to solids can be a big step. Moving from one texture to another in small increments makes the process easier, which is why those first pureed baby foods can be so watery that they don't seem much different from breast milk or formula.

FOOD TEXTURE PROGRESSION
Easier to Harder

LEVEL ONE
Kids learn to eat (or drink) more or less from the top of this list to the bottom. By the age of three, most kids are able to eat all the level-one foods.

Liquids
   thick to thin

Purees
   watery to pastelike
   creamy smooth to gritty
   thick and lumpy

Crunch and crumble (dry solids with uniform texture that dissolve
      when wet)

cheese curls	animal crackers
wagon-wheel crackers	pizza crust
dry cereal (Cheerios, Kix, and Chex)	veggie sticks
	zwieback
graham crackers	toast
Teddy graham crackers	bread sticks
saltines	

Moist solids (meltables to firm)

soft ripe fruit (banana)	pastina (tiny pasta, cooked soft)
canned fruits (mandarin oranges)	American cheese
	avocado
canned vegetables (green beans, kidney beans, etc.)	overcooked squash
pasta/macaroni (bigger sizes, cooked firm, are more difficult to eat)	

Soft solids

pancakes/waffles	bread
muffins	scrambled eggs
thin deli meats	

Lumpy or mixed texture foods/combination foods

lumps in thick puree to solids in a thin liquid (soup)

Note that many kids have problems with mixed-texture foods—a puree with lumps—like fruited yogurt. If a child struggles with these foods, increase textures gradually.

Bite-size foods

grilled cheese	cooked vegetables
chopped-meat sandwiches	fruit
mini waffles	

LEVEL TWO
Although there is wide variability, some kids don't completely master the skills to eat these foods until after age three.

Chewy solids

meat strips	raisins

Hard solids (These foods pose a choke risk for kids under the age of three.)

raw carrots	nuts
popcorn	hard candies

Pureed and Lumpy Foods

When kids struggle with food-texture progressions, even subtle texture differences matter. With stage one foods, some are watery and others pasty. It's easier to eat a thin, watery puree than to eat one that is dry and pasty. A drier, thicker texture requires more exaggerated swallowing movements in order to be effective. This is good if you want to strengthen the muscles (oral-motor skills) and bad if you want to maximize calories.

When every calorie matters, it's best to be careful about how much and which foods you thicken. Don't make every bite an ordeal.

After purees, kids typically move on to lumpy foods (mashed bananas) and chopped foods. Adding a thickener to purees with lumps or bits of other foods makes them easier to eat because it evens out the differences between the two textures.

Dry Foods

Dry, crunchy-textured food feels quite different from purees, and this can help a child focus on what to do next. Crumbly foods stimulate mouth muscles in new ways. Dry foods that quickly dissolve from saliva in the mouth are also called crunch-and-crumble foods (see the chart on page 150 for examples). These are hard enough to encourage biting, yet crumble quickly and, as a result, pose less risk for choking. You don't need teeth to eat these foods. In a practical sense, they melt in your mouth. This is a great feature when kids are first learning how to bite and chew.

Sometimes parents hold back on giving dry, crunchy foods such as dry cereal and crackers to picky eaters, but this can be a mistake. Some kids need the extra sensory experience from the dry foods to "wake up" the mouth.

At one year, Sarafina would put any food into her mouth,

chew it, and then spit it out. She was born one month early. Her parents thought she might just need some extra time. She didn't have any other problems related to her eating—no vomiting or gagging and no growth problems. Two months later, her parents worried that spitting out food was becoming a pattern, and they wondered why she was not swallowing.

The family was health-conscious and followed a low-carb diet. Since almost all crunch-and-crumble foods are carbohydrates, this meant that there were few of these "bad foods" in the house. When Sarafina's parents started giving her more crunch-and-crumble foods, she began to swallow more and spit out less. Within a month she had stopped spitting out food.

Combination Foods

Once kids have mastered crunch-and-crumble foods, most quickly move ahead to table foods. However, for some kids lumpy or mixed-texture foods present a struggle. Combination foods that mix together two or more textures can cause problems. Often a child can handle one or the other texture individually, but when two are combined, troubles arise. Soup made with a thin broth containing solid foods is the hardest to handle. The easiest to handle is a thick puree with lumps (such as a mashed ripe banana). The less difference there is between the textures, the easier the food will be to eat.

✕ *If your child is having problems with table foods, you may need to wait. Look for physical signs that your child is ready. Take a close look at how your child moves the tongue. Does it move from side to side? This is a critical step along the way to being able to bite and chew effectively. You can encourage this and other mature tongue movements (see page 53 for information about making mouth muscles stronger).*

For Jonah, learning to eat table foods was a slow process. At two, he ate only pureed baby foods. His growth was good; he walked but didn't talk. He also had a habit of grinding his teeth. A speech evaluation showed that he had abnormal tongue movement, which interfered with both his language and his eating.

With the help of a therapist, Jonah's parents learned how to fine-tune the progression of foods he was offered. The first food change was to thicken up the baby foods. Jonah wasn't thrilled with this and only a few foods were thickened. But once a day, Jonah did eat pasty, dry food that made his mouth muscles work harder. He was also given whistles and other toys that encouraged him to use his mouth in new ways. Along with this he was given strawberries and other soft fruit with a mesh feeder, which encouraged biting but avoided the risk of choking. Though normally used with younger children, it worked well for Jonah.

One day he was offered baby-food wagon wheels, a good crunch-and-crumble food that makes noise but dissolves fast. Being a typical two-year-old, Jonah refused. Luckily, his older sister was always ready to demonstrate the joys of eating these while Jonah looked on. Eventually he decided to give them a try.

And so it went, a long back-and-forth of encouraging Jonah to eat the next food on the list and waiting for him to go along with the idea. Some weeks he moved forward and other weeks he resisted. At one point he was eating Goldfish crackers ten times a day and refusing most other foods except milk—hardly a balanced diet.

Each step of increasing food textures happened slowly. After five months, Jonah was still refusing most table foods. Then, one day, he took a bite of his father's bagel. Amazingly, at a family gathering later that same day, Jonah ate one food after another, nonstop. He tried bread, crackers, cheese, dip, noodles, vegetables, fruit salad, cookies, ice cream—pretty much any food in sight was game. This openness to trying new foods continued at home, and went on for another two weeks. His parents were shocked at the change and initially concerned that the therapy had worked too well. But that stage, like the others, ended.

Finally, after six long months of therapy, Jonah was eating table foods, growing well, and no longer grinding his teeth. To the relief of many parents, the irksome habit of grinding teeth often stops when kids eat foods that require biting and chewing. The sensory explanation is that grinding teeth is a substitute for the stimulation they would otherwise get from chewing harder foods.

By one year of age, most kids are eating table foods. If your child doesn't move on to table foods as quickly as expected, consider his overall development. Often a delay in one area spills over into another area. For example, a child who is slow to crawl or walk is more likely to lag behind in eating skills. In the end, the goal is to keep the act of eating pleasant while encouraging a child to eat increasingly difficult foods.

✕ *If your child is not eating table foods by the first birthday, help is available. Kids eventually learn how to eat table foods, although some need extra time. Get a referral to early intervention or a feeding clinic.*

Meats

Meat, which requires extra chewing, is often a stumbling block for older toddlers who either can't or won't take the time to eat it. Some parents rely on commercial toddler foods because they provide the only form of meat that their child will eat. Generally the six-ounce dinners provide one ounce of meat—not a huge amount, although adequate for toddlers. Perhaps more important than the amount is the texture. If you read the ingredients carefully, you may see terms like "chicken, ground and formed."

✕ *If your child needs more protein or iron, check out other sources. Meat is a great source of protein and iron. If you are concerned that your child needs more of these nutrients, learn about the requirements in chapter 6, "How Much Nutrition Is Enough?"*

Once kids have mastered the skills needed to feed themselves table foods, they need to learn how much is enough. When kids overstuff their mouths with food, the best strategy is prevention: limit the amount of food offered at one time. If kids get upset, let them know that more food will be given after swallowing. Ask a child to open his mouth and show that he is ready for more.

Changing Food Textures

Thickeners change the consistency of food or drinks. Unless there's a problem eating table foods or drinking from a cup, most kids don't need them. But in situations where kids struggle to eat foods with new textures, thickeners can help to make eating or drinking easier. Thickeners tend to be a temporary crutch, something that helps kids transition to new textures.

HOW DO THICKENERS MAKE EATING EASIER?

Normally, when Allison ate chicken-stew toddler dinner, she gagged. Adding a thickener, which evened out the textural difference between the smooth gravy and the solid chunks of noodles, vegetables, and meat, enabled Allison to eat the stew without gagging.

When two-year-old Keith drank juice from an open cup, it dribbled down his chin. The therapist wanted him to develop jaw control and keep his lower lip on the cup rim. To help him, she added a thickener to the juice and stabilized Keith's chin while he drank from the cup. The changes helped and, as a result, there were no dribbles. A few tries later, Keith drank juice from a cup on his own, without thickener or chin support.

Thickeners don't have to be fancy. Commercial products are convenient but not necessary. There are also foods on the supermarket shelf that work. These are almost always less expensive and may be higher in calories, protein, and other nutrients. Adding a teaspoon of instant-pudding mix to milk thickens it. The following is a list of other foods off the supermarket shelf that can be used as thickeners:

FOR LIQUIDS

Pureed fruits or vegetables (5–11 calories per tablespoon)
Baby cereal (14 calories per tablespoon)
Instant pudding (20–25 calories per tablespoon)
Yogurt (8–16 calories per tablespoon)
Soft tofu (10 calories per tablespoon)

FOR SOLIDS

Baby cereal (14 calories per tablespoon)
Flaxseed meal* (25 calories per tablespoon)
Instant pudding (20–25 calories per tablespoon)
Potato flakes (11 calories per tablespoon)
Wheat germ* (27 calories per tablespoon)
Bread crumbs (22 calories per tablespoon)

---

*These fiber-rich, nutrient-dense foods should not be used in large amounts with babies or small children. Typically that means no more than one or two tablespoons per day.

You may prefer the convenience or the predictable consistency of commercial thickeners. These thickeners are commonly used with adults, which means that they are easy to find in pharmacies or medical-supply stores that cater to the elderly. But the same products are also used for kids.

Powders like Thick-It or Thick & Easy work best when used just before eating. If mixed ahead of time, the food or liquid may continue to set up. When mixed into drinks and poured into bottles or sippy cups, the mixture may become too thick to flow through the nipple or spout.

Thick-It
Milani Foods
2525 Armitage Avenue
Melrose Park, IL 60160
800-333-0003
www.precisionfoods.com

Thick & Easy
American Institutional Products, Inc.
2733 Lititz Pike
Lancaster, PA 17601

A newer product is now available. Simply Thick, a gel, does not break down over time. It stays the same consistency during a long feeding or when prepared ahead. It is often used as a thickener with breast milk. But it has drawbacks. It is the most costly product of its kind and, because this is a liquid, it dilutes the calorie concentration of food. It is not the best choice when every calorie counts.

Simply Thick
Phagia-Gel Technologies, LLC
1374 Clarkson Clayton Center
St. Louis, Missouri 63011
800-205-7115

Xanthum gum (which is used to make Simply Thick) is also available as a powder in health-food stores or online from www.bobsredmill.com.

Before commercial thickeners were available, baby rice cereal was often used. This is the least expensive thickener. However, you will need more of it. A rough rule of thumb is that you will need four times more rice cereal than you would need commercial thickener.

SPECIALTY FOODS/PRODUCTS:

Menu-Direct
Offers pureed foods that are shipped directly to your home
800-225-2610

Resource Thickened Juices
Available in handy individual-serving juice boxes
www.specialtyfoodshop.com

Dysphagia Resource Center
Lists various products for those with swallowing problems
www.dysphagia.com

Exactly how thick is thick enough? In some cases, therapists will specify the appropriate level of thickness with the terms "nectar," "honey," or "pudding." Commercial thickeners facilitate a precise degree of thickening and will specify how much to add to achieve these levels. But with some products, the final consistency depends on *when* a thickener is mixed into *which* food.

When it's important to get predictable consistency, the timing of when the thickener is added and when the food is eaten matters. Most thickeners are starch-based and these continue to set after mixing, making a food thicker the longer it sits. There is one exception to this—breast milk, which contains enzymes that break down starch. As a result, it's best to add a starch-based thickener to expressed breast milk just before using it; otherwise, the mixture will be thinner instead of thicker. This is the reason why some hospital nurseries add thickeners at the bedside.

The consistency of a food affects how easy it is to swallow, and for many children that is the main concern. For some, there are other considerations.

Adding a thickener to a food changes its calorie and fluid content. While in most cases this doesn't matter, when kids are underweight or at risk for dehydration these changes become more important. A pediatric dietitian can help you work out the details and avoid complications for any child with these risks.

Thickeners that contain protein or vegetable gums can bind some of the fluid and need to be used with care for kids who are at risk for dehydration.

In general, with picky eaters who need calories, wheat germ and other high-calorie foods are good choices. If a commercial thickener is used, the powders usually add calories while the gels lower them by displacing other liquids. This can be a problem for kids who are underweight and for whom every calorie counts.

Sensory Integration and Picky Eaters

George didn't like eating. But, then again, George didn't like a lot of things.

Outside, in his backyard, George didn't like walking barefoot on the grass. At the beach, George had to be carried: he didn't like to walk on sand.

George didn't like having his hair washed or cut. Nor did he like having his fingernails clipped. George was fussy about clothes. He didn't like wearing hats or shirts with tags.

He didn't like touching wet or sticky things with his hands. On the rare occasions when he touched a food that was sticky, George screamed to have his hands washed.

For therapists who work with kids who have sensory issues, children like George are familiar.

Sensitive kids who don't like having their hands dirty may refuse finger foods—especially those that are wet, sticky, gooey, or slimy. George did not like having messy hands. His mother thought he was just neat and tidy, but the occupational therapist who worked with him thought otherwise. In her report, the therapist described George as "sensory defensive." To help normalize his sensory reactions, she introduced George to a series of messy activities. Gradually he became more comfortable with having stuff on his hands and began to touch and bring food to his mouth.

Even though George brought food to his mouth, he didn't always eat it. Dry cereal and crackers were okay, but any soft, wet, or slimy food was not. Using specific oral-motor exercises, the occupational therapist essentially massaged George's mouth, inside and out. Doing this before mealtimes helped George to accept more foods. The exercises helped to desensitize his mouth, making many food textures more tolerable.

As he grew older, eating the dry cereal and crackers helped to "jump-start" him so that he ate soft foods more readily. George liked dry, crunchy foods. Giving these to him helped him to eat a wider variety of food textures. His mother learned little tricks for making foods drier and crunchier. Instead of zapping waffles in the microwave, she heated them in the toaster, and she always made his sandwiches with toasted bread. It all seemed to help. Over time, George grew less sensitive and began to accept food textures he had previously rejected, namely, anything soft, mushy, or slimy.

When a child is overly sensitive to food texture, feeling those textures in the mouth evokes sensations that are noxious and disturbing rather than interesting or pleasant. Sensory reactions to the tactile qualities of food range from overreactive to normal to underreactive.

Lauren was the polar opposite of George. The minute food entered her mouth, Lauren swallowed it. Because she was undersensitive, Lauren barely reacted to either the taste or the texture of the food in her mouth. She began having problems as an older baby whenever she was given foods with mixed textures. She could eat soft, chopped fruit without a problem, but if the fruit was mixed with a smooth food like yogurt, Lauren choked and gagged.

Lauren had no problem with soup as long as the solids were strained out. First she ate the soft solids and then drank the broth from the bowl or slurped it from a spoon. But if she tried to eat both solids and broth together in the same mouthful, it was a disaster. She choked, gagged, and burst into tears, often refusing to eat anything else for hours. The solution was simply to avoid mixed-texture foods until she was more mature. In time Lauren was able to eat everything. Along the way, her parents helped by reminding her to chew when they gave her foods that might cause a problem.

Lauren and George represent a simplistic model for understanding sensory reactions to the tactile properties of food. This simple model views reactions along a single continuum of extremes, from too much reactivity to too little reactivity. It is not the only model and it does not fit all children.

The stories about George and Lauren describe only the sensory issues related to eating. Therapists view sensory integration from a broader perspective. To learn more, the book *The Out-of-Sync Child* by Carol Kranowitz gives a more comprehensive description of sensory integration.

EXPANDING TASTE AND TEXTURE EXPERIENCES

Because children react differently to the taste, temperature, and texture of foods, it's important to recognize these sensitivities. They are both obstacles and pathways to expanding the variety of foods children will eat.

INTENSE FLAVORS

Some children naturally prefer foods with intense flavors. Others are so nonreactive to food that intensely flavored foods "wake up" a child's mouth and help him to focus on eating.

Here are a few examples of how to intensify food flavors:

Lemon/Lime Juice

Dip cut-up fresh fruit in lemon juice. It will add some zing and prevent fruits like apples from turning brown. Or add ¼ teaspoon to pureed food, such as fruit, to intensify the flavor.

Flavor Extracts

You can buy these in any grocery store. But if you want a deluxe version, try the Watkins brand. These are available online from www.therecipebox.com.

Italian Syrups

These sweet syrups come in a wide variety of flavors and can be added to food or medicine to make it more appealing. The grape and strawberry flavors are popular among kids who need to drink specialized formulas. They are normally used to flavor expresso-based beverages and are sold in coffee shops or online from www.kaldi.com.

Parmesan Cheese

A sprinkle of grated Parmesan or Pecorino Romano cheese adds a salty flavor that many kids enjoy. It also adds extra calcium and protein, making food more nutritious as well as tasty.

Pomegranate Molasses

This traditional food has a complex flavor that combines sweet and tart. A few drops added to water or food perks up the taste. It is available in Middle Eastern grocery stores or online from www.adrianascaravan.com (800-316-0820) or www.kalustyans.com (212-685-3451).

Salsa

Unlike ketchup, salsa counts as a legitimate vegetable serving. Use it as a dip or topping for scrambled eggs, potatoes, vegetables, beans, or rice. Buy mild salsa.

Seasoned Rice Vinegar

A small amount sprinkled over vegetables adds a pleasant zing. Look for this in the gourmet section of the supermarket or in an Asian grocery store.

Vinegar

Sprinkle vinegar and oil on cut-up vegetables (squash, peppers, potatoes, and onions) and roast in a hot oven (450 degrees) for 15 minutes. Both the high heat and the vinegar will intensify the flavors.

TEMPERATURE

When a child enjoys cold food temperatures, try freezing mini bagels, biscuits, muffins, bananas, and other soft fruits and vegetables. You can also make yogurt pops by mixing yogurt with fruit-juice concentrate.

BUILDING BRIDGES: STRATEGIES TO HELP CHILDREN ENJOY NEW FOODS

Heightened sensitivity to food textures and flavors can hamper a child's ability to eat age-appropriate foods. Often feeding specialists help children expand their skills and tolerance for new foods by making minute changes in texture or flavor. The approach is based on building bridges between the familiar and the new in small, incremental steps. While there are infinite variations, these are a few examples:

Texture-to-Texture

For a child who only eats smooth food, increase texture by sprinkling a gritty or drier food that does not require chewing (such as crushed cereal) into yogurt or other favorite smooth food. A number of foods can be used to increase the texture. They include baby cereal, crushed crackers, couscous, flaxseed meal, ramen noodles, and wheat germ.

To encourage a child to try a new texture, give it after the preferred texture. For example, give a child who prefers crunchy foods dry cereal before giving soft fruits.

Flavor-to-Flavor

For a child who seems stuck and eats only one or two flavors of pureed fruit, try to intensify the flavor with a small amount of lemon juice. Or slowly introduce a new flavor. If the preferred fruit is plain applesauce, add a spoonful of flavored applesauce to it, gradually shifting to more and more of the flavored applesauce.

Notice which flavors a child prefers and look for flavors that are similar. If a child drinks flavored milk, try the same flavor in a pudding.

Flavor-to-Texture

If a child likes cheese-flavored foods, use the sauce packet from a box of macaroni and cheese mix, substituting pastina or other small, easy-to-swallow pasta shape. Then gradually move up to bigger pasta shapes.

Regardless of which strategy is used, the idea is to make small changes that are noticeable but have some degree of familiarity. The new flavor or texture should be offered multiple times. Initially, children tend to eat less of the modified food. But as long as they eat some, they are making progress, and with consistent effort, generally continue to expand the number of foods they will eat.

While the concept of building bridges between familiar and new foods is straightforward, the reality of making it work, day after day, with very fussy eaters is challenging. There's no question that knowing when and how to nudge a child to go beyond what is comfortable can be difficult. Working with a professional who knows your child makes it easier.

Do

- Look for patterns in your child's food refusals. Keep them in mind when introducing new foods.
- Encourage your child to touch, smell, and be messy with food. Such experiences help children to eat better.
- Be cautious about giving your child foods with mixed textures; these are often more difficult to eat.
- Make it easier to learn how to drink from a cup. Offer your child sips of a shake or other thick drink from an open cup.
- Be prepared to expand the range of foods your child eats in small steps, if needed.

Don't

- Expect instant results when trying to expand a child's acceptance of new food textures or flavors.
- Assume your child dislikes water. Often the problem is due to the fact that it is more difficult to drink.
- Overwhelm your child with flavors or textures he is not ready to handle.
- Hesitate to seek help from a specialist if you suspect that your child's food refusals run deeper than those typical of a toddler.
- Blame yourself for your child's poor eating. Often children who don't progress with food textures have underlying sensitivities.

Family Influences

Preschooler and drama-queen-in-training Annalee learns fast. When Annalee hands her frazzled mother a frozen dinner to reheat, she rolls her eyes and adds a sarcastic "Yum." Her mother stares. Then she remembers her teenage son and realizes that Annalee is imitating her brother.

After babies learn the mechanics of how to eat table foods, they are ready for new challenges. Normally, sometime after a baby's first birthday, the focus shifts to the social exchanges around food. Kids discover there's more to learn from watching people than watching their plates.

Day after day, there are new lessons. One-year-old Rachel learns that when she drops her cracker, someone picks it up. Three-year-old Ben learns that if he makes a face while eating, his mother laughs. Whether inside or outside the home, with family or others, over time, the lessons add up to shaping a child's attitudes and behavior. Some of the lessons exacerbate picky eating or other difficult behavior. These learning experiences happen slowly and sometimes escape parent radar.

Tensions over Food

Now and then, emotional tensions run high and lead to distorted interactions over food. Situations in which this can happen include

1. Family problems that spill over into food dynamics
2. Expectations on what, why, or how kids eat
3. Kids with developmental delays
4. Family history of eating problems

FAMILY DYNAMICS

Sometimes a child gets caught up in a food drama that has less to do with the child and more to do with other family issues. Two-year-old Miranda was a beautiful child whose parents were upset by the news that she suffered from failure-to-thrive. They brought her to a clinic for evaluation and came home with a list of high-calorie foods. However, Miranda refused them.

Miranda's father was concerned about his daughter's poor growth. Each day, he asked his wife what Miranda had or had not eaten and suggested how she should feed their daughter. Often these discussions escalated, and they found themselves slamming doors and yelling at each other over the "right" way to feed her. While both parents doted on her, Miranda's poor eating had increased the tensions between them.

Despite her husband's veiled accusations, Miranda's mother felt she was not to blame. This was her second marriage and her third child. She sensed that family tensions had contributed to Miranda's poor eating.

Around the time that Miranda's mother needed to go back to work, she heard about a small, home-based day care that served home-cooked meals. When she visited, she mentioned Miranda's poor appetite. To her relief, the day-care provider remarked that she had helped other poor eaters. Hopeful, Miranda's mother sent her there.

In the new setting, Miranda tried new foods and ate more. Over the next few months, her growth improved, and finally it reached the normal range.

Sometimes, mealtimes become so emotionally charged that there's no recognizable resolution. One simple solution is a change of scenery. In Miranda's case, the day care provided a neutral environment. She went along with the new rules, expectations, and dynamics.

✕ *If you are unhappy with your child's eating behavior, watch her eat with others. Parents are often surprised at how differently a child behaves when eating in a new environment. If you can arrange it, watch how your child eats with others when you are not in sight. You might discreetly gain new insights.*

EXPECTATIONS—WHAT, WHY, AND HOW KIDS EAT

Children's appetites fluctuate with age, and sometimes parents feel their child isn't eating enough based on heightened expectations. In a national study of more than three thousand families, when asked whether their child was a picky eater the percentage of parents answering yes jumped from 19 percent for babies four to six months old to 50 percent for toddlers nineteen to twenty-four months old.

Yet even though many of these children were fussy about *what* they ate, apparently they were not fussy about *how much* they ate. Researchers reported that in a twenty-four-hour period, *all* the children took in the recommended number of calories or more.

In the same study, when asked how many times parents offered a new food before deciding that their child didn't like it, the majority answered three to five times. This is considerably less than the eight to fifteen times that social scientists recommend.

KIDS WITH DELAYS

As kids grow older it's best to shift the focus off a child's eating. This is harder to do when there is an obvious problem. Yet it remains an important goal.

As a baby, Paul had a swallowing problem, which made it harder for him to learn how to eat table foods. To help him, his three older brothers clapped every time Paul took a bite of food. This worked well early on. Paul enjoyed the attention and pushed himself to eat more difficult foods.

But a year later, when Paul was two, he was stuck. Even though he had learned *how* to eat table foods, at two and a half he still wanted his mother to spoon-feed him.

Paul's mother decided that their family meals might not be the best time to encourage him to feed himself. His brothers were too helpful.

During morning snack, while his brothers were at school, his mother coaxed Paul to pick up and use the spoon. Day after day he resisted. One day, just after she had helped Paul bring a spoonful of yogurt to his mouth, the phone rang. As she got up to answer it, she realized Paul had taken the spoon out of his mouth by himself. After that, she helped him bring the spoon to his mouth and let him take it out by himself. That was the turning point. From then on he made faster progress and soon began feeding himself without any help.

Regardless of whether or not there are feeding problems, children often eat best when they are not the focus of family attention.

FAMILY HISTORY OF EATING PROBLEMS

Before she became a mother, Eden had been a dancer who followed a strict diet and exercise regime. Taking care of her body became an obsession. At one point, she struggled with an eating disorder. Through counseling, she overcame it.

Years later, when pregnant, the eating issues resurfaced. It was hard to change her habits. For support, she saw a nutritionist about adding extra fat, carbohydrates, calories, and vitamins. But she didn't like the nutritionist and had a hard time following the recommendations. She was relieved when she gave birth to a healthy daughter and no longer needed to agonize over what she ate.

As her daughter, Hannah, grew older, Eden saw issues around food flare up at various stages. With each episode, Eden struggled. There were days when she didn't want to deal with it anymore.

These incidences reopened old wounds and eventually increased tensions with her husband. With food, Eden described herself as "disciplined." Her husband described her as "rigid."

Eden found it hard to balance her food preferences with the foods Hannah liked to eat. She rarely ate with her daughter. After a while, it became easier just to give her daughter a liquid supplement. This led to Hannah refusing to eat solid foods.

Hannah's growth was normal, but her eating skills and behavior around food were not. Eden finally came to terms with the situation and decided to do something. She talked to the doctor about a referral to a feeding clinic for Hannah. Once there, she talked to the social worker and joined a mothers' group.

✕ *If you have a history of eating problems, don't assume they will go away. Researchers at Stanford University found that mothers with a past or present eating disorder fed their children on a less regular schedule, used food for nonnutritive purposes, and demonstrated a significantly higher concern for their daughters' weight.*

The researchers suggested that their female children might be at greater risk for the later development of an eating disorder.

Whatever the problem, if parents are too focused on food, they may miss the bigger issue. When the tensions around food arise, step back and look at the social dynamics.

WHAT TO DO WHEN KIDS DISCOVER FOOD AS A WAY TO GET ATTENTION

- Cut down the emotional "noise" around eating. Because young children enjoy drama, it's best not to overreact to a child's behavior around food.
- Use nonfood ways to give a child attention. Read a book, go for a walk, cuddle, or talk.
- Give kids choices. This helps defuse the power battles that often arise with toddlers.
- Avoid constant battles over food. One way to do this is to set reasonable limits and be consistent. Generally, parents control where, when, and what.
- Allow kids to say no to food.
- As kids grow older, encourage them to assume more responsibility for their food choices.

Shaping Food Habits

Among people from different parts of the world, the definitions of acceptable and not acceptable foods vary greatly. Most Americans would not eat snakes, dogs, or horses. Likewise, people from other cultures would not eat cows or pigs. Most of us learn the rules about which foods are proper and improper during childhood. Often these attitudes are deep-seated and difficult to change.

I have found patterns based on the cultural backgrounds of

my clients. When I ask parents to describe their toddlers' likes and dislikes, most list meats as unpopular. But often my Hispanic clients, especially those from the Dominican Republic, report something different. Their kids love meat, especially chicken legs and steak. In one interview, I incredulously asked a mother, "Chicken legs?" "Oh, yes," she answered. "My sister gave him his first chicken leg at eight months and he has loved them ever since."

I learned a lesson from this conversation and others like it. There's a benefit to introducing adult foods early.

Researchers have long recognized that many children go through a stage of neophobia—fear of new foods—between eighteen and twenty-four months of age. This is a time when kids are most likely to say no to food, which means that often the best time to expose kids to new foods is *before* this stage.

Parents often rely on special "baby foods" available for older babies and toddlers. Years ago, baby-food manufacturers were less imaginative. They created simple purees, which babies used for a few months. Because the array of baby-food choices has expanded, there's a tendency to prolong the time that young children and adults eat different foods. I don't think this is good.

Many parents assume that as kids get older they will be more open to trying new foods. But the evidence doesn't support this. One study found that kids who enjoyed a variety of foods at age two were more likely to still enjoy a variety of foods at age four. And the kids who didn't eat a variety of foods at two weren't any more likely to do it by age four.

If you want to influence your child's food choices, keep these suggestions in mind:

- **Be a good role model.**
  Study after study shows there's a link between what parents and their children eat. One found that mothers who

drank milk had five-year-old daughters who drank more milk and fewer soft drinks than mothers who didn't drink milk.

• **"Do as I do" is more effective than "Do as I say."**
When parents tell kids how to eat better by controlling their food choices, it doesn't work as well as being a good example. In fact, several studies show that there are risks in trying to control what kids eat.

• **Make healthy foods available and convenient.**
As children grow older, researchers report that they are more likely to eat fruits and vegetables that are washed, cut, and ready to eat. Make a list of fruits and vegetables you want to keep on hand. If you need ideas or recipes, check out the 5 A Day program on the www.cdc.gov Web site.

• **Expose kids to a variety of foods—the earlier the better.**
There's an assumption that kids learn to like a greater variety of foods as they grow older. Unfortunately, few studies have actually looked at this. One small study (reported in the November 2002 issue of the *Journal of the American Dietetic Association*) followed seventy children over a five-year period, up to age eight. They concluded that foods introduced after the age of four were more likely to be disliked than liked.

• **Eat together.**
When I advise mothers to sit and eat with their children, most look at me as though I am daft. I know young children need lots of attention when they eat. Yet if parents only watch and don't set an example, meals spiral downward. Kids eat better when they watch others eat and eat worse if adults watch them too intently while they eat.

- **If your child refuses the foods you have offered, WAIT.**
  When a younger child refuses food, a good response is to wait. Don't overreact, jump up, and get another food. Sometimes kids don't know what or if they want to eat. Give them time to decide, and they may eat what is in front of them.

- **If your child screams for food in the supermarket, don't give in.**
  If you give in, it only increases the chances that your child will do it again.

- **Avoid buying junk food to keep your child happy.**
  Parents naturally want to keep their children happy, and buying candy bars, soft drinks, and other low-nutrient foods is often an easy way do it. Look for healthier ways to keep your child happy.

Parents are not the only ones trying to influence children's food choices. Advertisers spend millions of dollars to entice children to demand goodies. Considering the epidemic rise of obesity and food-related health problems, it makes sense to take preemptive steps to prevent food problems *before* they start. Restricting junk foods and encouraging healthy eating seems like a no-brainer. The question is, does it really work?

Dr. Leann Birch at Pennsylvania State University has spent years doing research on eating behavior in young children. She has explored two strategies that parents often use to help children eat healthier. One is restricting children's access to unhealthy foods and the other is exerting pressure on children to eat foods that are "good for them."

In her research, parents were questioned on the degree of restriction they placed on their children's access to "unhealthy" snack foods. She then looked at how their children behaved when they were given access to these foods in settings without parents present to restrict their choices.

After doing several studies, Birch concluded that the restrictions actually *increased* the amount of the unhealthy foods eaten. The research also suggests that a similar paradoxical effect occurs when parents pressure kids to eat certain foods.

When I met four-year-old Casey and her mother, I thought of Dr. Birch's research. Casey and her mother had constant food battles. At preschool Casey was fine, but at home she was not. Casey's mother had strong feelings about junk foods and made a point to restrict any that came into the house. The problem was that Casey knew that the foods were there and that she couldn't have them. This made her want them more.

For the first half of the school year, Casey's mother continued to report food showdowns with her daughter. When her frustrations peaked, she met with Casey's teacher to ask for help. But after their meeting, Casey's mother realized that her daughter didn't have problems with food in school. Through counseling,

---

KEYS TO A HEALTHY FEEDING RELATIONSHIP WITH BABIES AND TODDLERS

- Be smart about giving help. Balance a child's need for assistance with the need for encouragement.
- Expect your child's developmental skills to spill over into eating.
- Offer appropriate food, formula, or breast milk. Then allow your child to initiate and guide feeding interactions.
- Trust and support your child's ability to self-regulate calories. Unless a doctor suggests otherwise, base feedings on your child's signs of hunger and satiety.

SOURCE: Adapted from the Start Healthy Feeding Guidelines for Infants and Toddlers, *Journal of the American Dietetic Association*, March 2004.

she learned to set reasonable limits with her daughter and their food battles subsided.

Casey's story and the Birch research findings show that caring parents need to be smart in their approach to limiting unhealthy foods. It's easy to go overboard.

For younger babies and toddlers, parents can follow the guidelines from Start Healthy. Underlying all the guidelines is the idea of a division of responsibility between parent and child. A parent takes responsibility for what, when, and where the child eats. The child decides whether or not to eat and how much.

Beyond Family Influence

After watching a television ad, a child tells her mother that she wants to celebrate her third birthday at an Applebee's restaurant. Over time, kids encounter food messages from ever-widening social circles that extend outward from the family to neighbors, church, school, community, and, to the dismay of many—the media.

In 1933, Popeye, the spinach-chomping sailor, appeared in short films that were shown in theaters across the country. The Popeye cartoons did more than entertain; they inspired millions of Americans to eat spinach. During the 1930s, spinach consumption in the United States jumped 33 percent.

Today, the tradition continues in a new form: advertisers use cartoon characters to sell sweet snacks and other products to children. There are *Dragon Tales* and *Cat in the Hat* fruit snacks, Elmo juice and cookies, and *Scooby-Doo* and *Flintstones* vitamins. Food advertising with or without cartoon characters accounts for roughly half of the ads targeted to children. Which foods are children being encouraged to eat? Candy (32 percent), cereal (31 percent), and fast food (9 percent).

The Center for Science in the Public Interest and others view food advertising to children as a problem. In addition to health issues, there is the idea of fair play. When watching television, children under the age of six can't distinguish between ads and regular programming. Yet children as young as two recognize and often request foods by brand name.

Public health programs promoting healthy foods can't compete with for-profit food companies. Advertising is expensive and the food industry is the second largest advertiser in the U.S. economy. Examples of the advertising budgets in 2004 of the largest food companies include Nabisco cookies and crackers ($100 million), Snickers candy bars ($45 million), Coke ($138 million), and McDonald's ($318 million).

✕ *Turn off the TV and your child will see fewer food commercials. The American Academy of Pediatrics recommends no TV or videos for children under the age of two and suggests limiting screen media time for older children to one to two hours of quality programming per day.*

Food messages aimed at children take many forms. In her book *Food Politics: How the Food Industry Influences Nutrition and Health*, Marion Nestle, a professor at New York University, writes:

Places to advertise to children are limited only by the marketer's imagination. Food companies put their logos on toys, games, clothing, and school supplies. They produce magazines, sponsor clubs, distribute coupons, buy product placements in movies, obtain celebrity endorsements, and even add their logos to baby bottles and Macy's Thanksgiving Day balloons.

Examples of food-brand logos on math and reading books for preschoolers and young children are: *Hershey's Kisses Counting Book, Kellogg's Froot Loops Counting Fun Book, Reese's Pieces Counting Board Book, M&M's Chocolate Candies Math, Cheerios Counting Book, Twizzler's Percentage Book, Skittles Riddles Math,* and *Sun-Maid Raisins Play Book.*

One justification for using food-brand logos on educational materials is that it increases the fun factor in learning and the food message is minimal. Not everyone agrees. One mother who battled with other family members to limit high-sugar foods in her house complained when a therapist used an Oreo cookie puzzle to teach shapes. After the therapy session, her child wanted Oreo cookies.

✕ *To counteract the influence of food advertising, learn more. A well-documented article entitled "Food Advertising and Marketing Directed at Children and Adolescents in the U.S.," from the University of Minnesota, gives a good overview. This "open access" article is available online at www.ijbnpa.org.*

It's hard to make an argument that any single food, regardless of sugar, fat, or calorie count, poses a health risk. Any food in moderation is safe. The problem is that when it comes to moderation with food, there's ample evidence that Americans are not doing well. The question becomes, do children need special protection?

Many believe they do. The American Psychological Association has urged lawmakers to place tighter restrictions on kids' ads. The American Academy of Pediatrics and other health-care groups support this.

Family Meals and Traditions

As her mother left the drive-through bank-teller window, three-year-old Tiffany asked, "What, no French fries?" At first, the question made her mother laugh; then, after thinking it over, it made her uncomfortable. Maybe that fast-food drive-through with her daughter was happening too often.

Millions of parents use fast foods to solve the daily dilemma of what to feed the kids. In the last thirty years, American children's fast-food consumption has increased sixfold. Three out of four children eat fast foods at least once a week.

National surveys show that 80 percent of American families want to have meals together, but the reality is that only half actually manage to do it. It's hardly surprising that fast foods have grown so popular. Researchers note other changes in the way Americans eat:

- **Snacks are popular with adults and kids.**
  In one adult survey, 24 percent skipped a meal in favor of snacks and 10 percent grazed all day. National surveys have reported a rise in the number of calories children consume through snacks rather than meals.

- **More Americans eat on the go—especially in the car.**
  Sales of portable meals and snacks are up. Food bars are especially popular.

- **Many Americans eat while watching television.**
  One survey found that 42 percent of meals eaten at home by middle-school children were consumed in front of the TV. When we eat on the go or in front of the television, we disconnect ourselves from food as well as from people. This has social and psychological ramifications.

- **Eating out is popular.**
  Lack of time and ideas for what to make for family meals makes it easier than ever to eat out. But research shows that the nutritional quality of foods eaten outside the home drops while the calories go up.

- **When families eat together, they may not eat the same foods.**
  Many families suffer a generational food gap, with children and adults eating different foods.

  Often when young children are neophobic and fear new foods, while their parents are at the opposite extreme. Neophilia—a love of the new—is a common attitude among adventurous adults who enjoy new and exotic foods. Lots of families resolve the conflict by eating together, but eating differently: the kids eat macaroni and cheese while the adults eat sushi.

  In the long run, it's easier to eat together when everyone eats the same foods. Try to minimize generational food gaps whenever possible.

Putting together meals day after day can be wearing, especially when kids fuss and whine. Yet making the effort to have family meals has countless benefits. How do families make it work? A book that includes recipes and stories on how families can connect through food is *Back to the Table: Reunion of Food and Family* by Art Smith.

Here are some other ideas on how to make family meals work:

Solve the problem of what to cook.
- Freeze whole meals in advance. Spaghetti sauce, chili, casseroles, and pesto are popular.
- If you are not much of a cook, find five simple recipes you

can make. Buy all the ingredients ahead of time so they are ready when you need them.

- If you enjoy cooking, you need to be more organized to do it with young children underfoot. Collect twenty to thirty recipes that are easy to moderate in difficulty and make a list of the ingredients. Compile it into one packet so that you don't need to go through your cookbooks before grocery shopping.
- When time is limited, take shortcuts. Use frozen and pre-pared foods for part or all of the meal. Or order pizza and make a salad.

Get help.
- Adults can pick up takeout food to bring home.
- Three- and four-year-olds can help with simple chores like setting the table, tearing lettuce for salads, unloading gro-cery bags, making sandwiches, and putting things in the trash.

Keep meals uncomplicated.
- One family microwaves potatoes and tops them with canned chili and cheese.
- Another sets out plates and places whatever food is available on them. Sometimes it's fruit, bread, cheese, and sliced meat.
- Keep basic ingredients for a chef's salad ready in the refrig-erator: lettuce, hard-boiled eggs, deli meats, cheese, beans, and veggies.

All meals count. If dinner doesn't work, try breakfast. This is an especially good time for young children who tend to be hun-grier early in the day.

Use common sense. Food choices are personal and varied. Do what works for your family.

In the end, family meals are about more than food. When the family sits and eats together—whether it's takeout, leftovers, or home-cooked—kids benefit. Mealtimes matter. Research shows that kids who eat with their families do better in several areas:

- They make healthier food choices.
- They have a lower risk for eating disorders.
- They are more motivated at school.
- They form better relationships.
- They are less likely to use alcohol or drugs.

Keep all these benefits in mind when schedules are tight and the traditional sit-down, home-cooked meals aren't realistic. Even if the food you eat is not perfect, the simple act of sharing food with those you love is worthwhile.

Do
- Consider the influence of family dynamics on your child's eating habits.
- Expect your child's age and development to affect her eating.
- Make healthy foods convenient and available.
- Make it a habit to eat together as a family.

Don't
- Assume your own eating behavior doesn't influence your child.
- Allow your child to overhear discussions about her eating.
- Have battles over food with your child.
- Openly react to your child's eating or not eating.
- Ignore media influences on your child's food preferences.

Mealtime Do's and Don'ts

The grandmother of a picky eater once said to me with a sigh, "When I raised my own children, things were easier. It was simple. I put out food and they ate it. Why doesn't that work anymore?"

The basics of eating haven't changed: we still eat to survive. Yet a new landscape of food choices, combined with the distractions of modern life, has changed our relationship to food. Our grandmothers couldn't buy yogurt in plastic squeeze pouches, or drive through a fast-food restaurant on the way to a soccer game. These new options change what, how, and sometimes why we eat—especially for kids.

With the ever-growing number of junk foods and food-related health problems, it's easy and understandable to worry so much about "what" a child eats that you forget about "how." But part of the picky-eating solution is looking beyond the quality and quantity of the food a child eats to the dynamics around mealtime.

Researchers cite links between early eating experiences and

eating problems later in life. Considering ways to improve meal-times for young children encourages healthier lifelong eating.

What Doesn't Work at Mealtimes—and Why

To avoid some common mealtime pitfalls with your child,

DON'T
- offer giant portions.
- allow daylong grazing.
- force food.
- use distractions.
- offer bribes, punishments, and rewards.
- encourage long mealtimes.
- let kids throw food.
- react emotionally to food refusals.
- reward food refusals.

DON'T OFFER GIANT PORTIONS

Even though large portions have been shown to encourage overeating in overweight children, they actually don't help under-weight children eat more. In fact, offering large portions tends to overwhelm small, young children. More than once, I have watched children refuse big helpings and only moments later happily eat the same food in smaller portions.

One mother gave her frail, underweight two-year-old daugh-ter, Amanda, a bowl filled with bite-sized crackers. Amanda turned up her nose and shook her head. We took the bowl away and counted out three crackers on her tray. One by one, Amanda ate them. When I asked her if she wanted more, she said yes. She said yes for three more rounds before she stopped.

BIG BENEFITS

Encouraging kids to ask for more has benefits that go beyond eating:

- Teaches a healthy social interaction
- Encourages speech and self-expression
- Gives a child a sense of empowerment

DON'T ALLOW DAYLONG GRAZING

Look at the snacks and drinks your child consumes during the day. Too many usually means kids won't be hungry for meals. Be sure to count everything—the sips of juice as well as the bites of solid foods.

Drinking liquids is easier than chewing solids, especially for young children. Among underweight children seen in feeding clinics, it's not uncommon to find them sipping juice and other high-calorie drinks all day long. There are reports of children drinking a quart or more of juice a day.

Common sense suggests that drinking extra calories would help an underweight child. After all, calories are calories. But those who work in specialty clinics for such children find that the habit of daylong drinking increases the odds that a child will be a poor eater. So, if your child is thirsty, offer water.

DRINKS ADD UP

And dull appetites—even wholesome ones. What's too much? Each day, no more than
    4–6 ounces of juice.
    32 ounces of milk.

DON'T FORCE FOOD

Pushing food on kids doesn't work. The harder parents push, the less likely a child will be a good eater. When I talk to parents who report they have pressured or forced a child to eat, I ask for their permission to playact. I pick up a spoon and hold it to their lips. Ignoring startled expressions, I ask parents how they feel. Do they want to push me away? As they nod yes, I warn that this instinctive reaction starts early. A child feels the same way.

Never force-feed a child. Children who have been pushed or forced to eat learn to hate eating.

DON'T USE DISTRACTIONS

Distractions vary—but unexpected interruptions easily get kids off track. Barking dogs, ringing phones, noisy neighbors, yelling siblings, and other mealtime interruptions can prevent children from eating well. Of course, there's only so much you can control, but too much noise or stimulation can interrupt a child's eating and bring a quick end to a meal. If growth is a concern, make the effort to reduce the chaos of life during mealtimes.

There's another category of distractions—intentional ones we offer to make eating easier, or so it seems. These include eating while

- watching television
- playing with toys at the table
- riding in the car
- playing games

The problem is not that these distractions don't work at all. It's that they work at the beginning, but over time diminish a child's interest in eating. Bringing children's attention to the food in front of them helps them connect the act of eating with the subtle cues of hunger and satiety. Practice helps kids recognize when they have eaten too much or too little.

Limit the times a child eats while doing something else. Anything that disconnects a child's attention from eating potentially interferes with establishing good eating habits.

TV FOOD ADS DO MORE THAN DISTRACT

They send a powerful, unhealthy message.

- Food manufacturers are the second largest advertisers in the U.S. economy.
- TV ads account for 75 percent of their advertising dollars.
  What foods are advertised? The top three:
  > breakfast cereals
  > candy and gum
  > soft drinks
  At the bottom: fruits and vegetables
- Food marketers estimate that American children begin asking for name-brand products by the age of two.

DON'T OFFER BRIBES, PUNISHMENTS, AND REWARDS

Desperate parents of picky eaters sometimes go to amazing lengths to get kids to eat. They promise rewards, treats, toys, and even trips. The old line "If you don't eat your peas, no dessert" has been inflated to "If you don't drink your milk, no video games" or "no trip to Disneyland."

Like distractions, rewards and punishments work in the short run. Usually at first, a child unhappily stuffs in a few more bites, but in the long run, things get worse. The child's motivation to eat has more to do with the social dynamics around eating and less to do with feeling hungry.

Clever children who sense their parents' desperation hold out for bigger rewards. I once worked with a mother whose child refused to eat unless she took her to McDonald's.

Common advice is to not use food as a reward or a punishment. Avoid saying "*If* you eat your peas, you can have dessert." This teaches a child that sweets are a reward for eating vegetables—not a great message.

DON'T ENCOURAGE LONG MEALTIMES

When meals are unpleasant and last longer than thirty minutes, something may need to change. Unless a child has physical problems involving the mechanics of eating, long mealtimes are usually a sign of putting too much energy in trying to get a child to eat and children taking advantage.

Avoid power struggles over food. Coaxing, coddling, games, and threats generally lead to unpleasant mealtimes.

One father simply would leave food out for his son and let him wander back to take more bites, then run off to play, then come back to the table again. A nibble here and there, for up to two hours after a meal, never added up to the calories he needed for normal growth.

Keeping mealtimes short is a simple way to avoid trouble. Put out all the food at once, limit interruptions during the meal, and put the food away after thirty minutes are up. Within a few days kids will learn to eat when food is served.

DON'T LET KIDS THROW FOOD

When a child throws food, it is a sign that eating is over. Calmly remove food in a matter-of-fact way. This prevents a child from using food to gain attention.

Cherie, a newly adopted eighteen-month-old baby, was struggling with life in a new home. She cried for hours and threw her food. Her stressed-out parents asked for help. I suggested that the next time Cherie threw her food, her parents should say "Bye-bye, food" and immediately take it away. It's important to do this without anger. The idea of taking food away is not to punish the child but to give a clear message that if food is thrown, it goes away. Timing also matters. The food needs to be taken away quickly to give clear feedback.

After two days, Cherie stopped throwing food. Her mom added that their first episode of "Bye-bye, food" happened with yogurt, a food she knew Cherie liked. I suspect this helped. Her mom recalled, "I'll never forget the look on her face when I threw her yogurt away."

In some instances, kids throw food as a last resort. Has your child given earlier signs that he no longer wants to eat? You may be able to prevent food throwing before it even happens. Look for and accept early signs that your child is finished eating.

DON'T REACT EMOTIONALLY TO FOOD REFUSALS

When parents get upset or angry with a child for not eating, it sends precisely the wrong message. I once witnessed a frustrated mother scolding her son for not eating his peas, telling him, "You are a bad boy and I won't love you if you don't eat your peas." Children need to eat for their own well-being, not to please or displease a parent.

It is important to give a child the time he needs to learn to recognize his own body signals of hunger and fullness. Adolescents and adults with eating disorders often confuse physiological sensations with emotional feelings. Researchers believe the pattern starts in childhood.

Young children crave love and attention from parents and parents need to give lots of it—but it's best to leave food out of it. Read a book together. Give hugs and kisses. Sing, smile, and respond to your child. Find other ways to demonstrate your love and give your child attention.

Sometimes parents need to plan ahead to avoid getting upset about a child's food rejections. One mother spent hours cooking homemade foods that her young daughter usually refused to eat. Day after day, the mother found herself eating the rejected foods. This added to her frustration. At my suggestion, she began using convenience foods, which reduced the emotional tension and helped this mother feel less angry and resentful when her daughter refused to eat. To her surprise, after a few weeks her daughter began to eat better.

DON'T REWARD FOOD REFUSALS

As babies grow into toddlers, the responsibility for eating shifts away from the parent to the child. Child feeding experts have mapped out the lines of "who" does "what" at this age. It's the parents' responsibility to provide appropriate food, and the child's to decide whether or not to eat.

When your toddler refuses pancakes, don't offer waffles. Offering a new food after the first food is rejected only rewards your child's refusal. It teaches her "If I say no, I might get something better." Parents who do this regularly soon become short-order cooks, offering one thing after another in the hope that their children will eventually eat something.

When a child refuses the first offering, being firm about not providing new foods will help him be less fussy and eat more. For parents who don't mind making three different meals, I suggest putting the energy into making one big banquet. It's better to offer a child choices at the beginning of a meal.

What Does Work at Mealtimes

To improve mealtime dynamics,

Do
- Set clear and consistent limits.
- Support independence.
- Allow a child to express preferences.
- Create schedules and routines.
- Establish a place for eating.
- Provide good role models.
- Include mellow-out time.
- Offer easy-to-eat foods.
- Have fun.
- Try reverse psychology.
- Practice patience.

SET CLEAR AND CONSISTENT LIMITS

Young children need limits, even though they may test those limits over and over. Consistency is a cardinal rule; otherwise children learn that if they push hard enough, they will get their way. Consistency is hard for parents to maintain day in and day out. But don't let your child wear you down. It is important to be firm in setting limits so that "no" really means "no."

Kids are smart. Setting limits consistently but not too harshly takes practice. Parents can gain skills and confidence from watching someone who has a firm but gentle hand with children.

One day I watched a preschool teacher repeatedly set limits on the out-of-bounds behavior of an intensely active three-year-old named Ralph. Soon after coming into the classroom, Ralph took all the books out of the bookcase and refused to let any of the other children look at them. The teacher did not scold him, but she made it clear that he could not take all the books for himself; he had to share. Ralph pouted, huffed, and walked away from the group. With each activity, Ralph behaved provocatively until the teacher stopped him, again and again. But each time he recovered more quickly.

At snack time, Ralph smiled when offered a choice of animal crackers or applesauce. He insisted on getting specific animals, but the teacher ignored his requests, telling him, "It's okay. They all taste the same." He behaved well until the end of snack, when he ran away from the table clutching a cracker. The teacher went after him and said, "If you want the cracker you have to eat it at the table." "No, no, no," he screeched, "I want the cracker here." The teacher took the cracker away and said, "I'm sorry, but you cannot eat the cracker here." Ralph went off sulking, but he soon rejoined the group playing kickball, which he loved. At the end of the session, Ralph gave his teacher a big smile.

There's a difference between what children want and what they need. Ralph had a hard time knowing how to behave in the classroom. It was a very different world from the one he had at home. His teacher recognized Ralph's struggle. She consistently made the rules clear. Eventually Ralph accepted the classroom rules, learned how to play with the other children, and enjoyed going to preschool.

Kids are cute, charming, and persistent, all of which help them wear parents down. But setting appropriate limits is important. The best way to do it is nicely, consistently, and firmly.

It is not always clear why children are provocative. Mealtimes are often unhappy when children intentionally misbehave. Although rules are necessary, try to limit the number of battles by making as few rules as possible, especially for toddlers.

To avoid being a constant block to your child's desires, use other parenting techniques, such as redirecting her attention. If a child insists on orange juice when only apple juice is available, try making up a story about apple juice, or explain how drinking any liquid quenches thirst, or talk about some upcoming exciting activity. Soon she will forget she wanted orange juice.

SUPPORT INDEPENDENCE

Young children alternate between wanting help and wanting independence, needing support one minute and limits the next. To make it work, parents need to be flexible and authoritative. This is not easy, but a good rule is to give children help only when they need it.

One day, three-year-old Tyler began asking his mother, Rachel, to spoon-feed him. She was puzzled. Tyler had been feeding himself for more than a year. Why the change?

Rachel was in the last trimester of pregnancy when Tyler first asked her to feed him. My guess is that Tyler sensed an impending change in his life and that being spoon-fed made him feel more secure. It's common for kids to regress when a new sibling comes into the house. Rachel understood Tyler's need for extra support, so she fed Tyler when he asked her to, but she put limits on her efforts. When he started fidgeting more and eating less, she stopped feeding him and encouraged him to do so on his own.

Mealtimes worked out for Rachel and Tyler. But more than once I've seen situations where they did not. Parents who are worried about a child's poor growth are likely to get into trouble by feeding a child who is able to do it on his own. Although spoon-feeding two- and three-year-olds is not unheard of, parents should be wary.

Often, adults and children have different agendas. An adult wants to get food into a child, while the child wants to play and get attention. This scene plays out in different ways. If you feel frustrated or find that your efforts are unproductive (i.e., your child is not eating), then stop.

One way to gauge whether your child needs you to help or to set limits is to step back and think about his behavior in a broader context than mealtimes. How is he behaving in other areas of his life? Is he more clingy than usual? Has his nap schedule changed? You may find it's easier to recognize when your child needs help or limits in these areas.

ALLOW A CHILD TO EXPRESS PREFERENCES

Give your child choices at each meal. This gives kids some control and encourages active participation. You don't want to make a child feel passive—like a container that needs to be stuffed with food.

Your job is to decide what foods are offered and your child's job is to decide what and whether or not to eat. Include foods that you know she likes as well as ones you want her to eat. But encourage kids to try new foods on their own. Say something like, "Look, we have broccoli. Oh, you don't want any? Okay, it's here if you decide to try it. It's delicious."

Of course, encouraging kids to make their own food choices is not the end of the story. Once parents open the door to kids expressing food likes and dislikes, there are new challenges.

CHOICES

Give kids choices such as:

- What foods do you want to eat *first*?
- Which plate, spoon, or cup do you want to use?
- Do you want this cracker or that cracker?

Five-year-old Jackson liked to make his younger brother laugh. One day he said "Yuk" and made a face at the food on his plate. His brother broke out with a howling laugh. With such a great audience, Jackson repeated his act and soon stopped eating more foods. After a few months of this, he had a very short list of foods he would eat.

His parents wondered how many vitamins Jackson was missing and how long this stage would last. Although worried about their son, they were unsure of how to help him. Finally, they decided to put limits on his constant "yuk" reactions to food. They made a rule: Jackson couldn't say he didn't like a food unless he tasted it. This became a bit of a game, with his parents offering new, enticing foods and Jackson exploring a minimalist approach to food tasting: his solution was a tiny lick. Whenever a new food was put on the table, everyone watched Jackson's reaction, his younger brother waiting for a good laugh and his parents hopefully anticipating that with the right food or right situation, Jackson's eating would start to improve.

His parents never forced him to eat, but Jackson knew they wanted him to eat more foods. Eventually he did. But it didn't start at home. He did it at school, where no one was interested in what foods he ate or did not eat. Gradually that behavior transferred to home.

CREATE SCHEDULES AND ROUTINES

If you provide regular times and places for eating, you'll set the stage for better mealtimes. Kids learn that there is a special time for food, and, as a result, they are less likely to fuss about it.

Adam's parents were graduate students living on campus. Adam's mom had to juggle school, part-time work, and family, which meant she fed Adam at different times and in different places from one day to the next. Some days Adam ate well and on others he barely touched his food. Because his growth was normal, it seemed that Adam was able to adapt to the irregular schedule. Not all children do as well.

One of the advantages of having routines is that the structure helps us recognize when a child eats better.

- Some children eat better with other family members while others eat well only for Mom.
- Often a child will consistently eat best at a particular meal. If a child always eats a good breakfast, it makes sense to offer more food then.

Timing of meals also affects a child's appetite. Occasionally, professionals who work with picky eaters recommend spacing meals three or four hours apart with no snacks or drinks (other than water) in between. The idea is to ensure that a child will be hungry when food is finally offered. One of the problems cited for children with poor appetites is that they have not learned to recognize or feel hunger. Stretching out the time between meals creates stronger hunger cues.

ESTABLISH A PLACE FOR EATING

Encourage eating in a particular place. The classic setting is at the table or in the high chair. This helps teach children that if they want to eat, they must do it in this place. It's a good idea to get kids into this habit early—before a child learns how to walk.

Another advantage to having a place for eating is that it builds an association. Over time, a child learns "When I am in this place, it is time to eat." Having a place that is used only for eating makes the association stronger. Parents who want to do this in a small space can achieve similar results by using other "only at eating time" conditions, such as playing particular music, using a table-cloth or placemats, or in some way creating a distinctive mealtime environment.

PROVIDE GOOD ROLE MODELS

Having meals with young children can be messy and demanding. Yet eating together has both long- and short-term benefits. Kids are great imitators. If you set a good example, your child will learn from watching you. Older siblings and other children are big influences too. Often children will eat more or try new foods in preschool when they sit with others who are good eaters. Countless mothers report their children trying a new food after seeing an older child eating it.

LOOK FOR GOOD ROLE MODELS

Being away from home makes it easier to introduce kids to new foods. Take advantage of this. Plan to visit friends, relatives, or places that inspire your child to eat better or try new foods.

For mothers on weight-loss diets, eating with a picky toddler can be a struggle. It's hard to face the temptation of high-calorie foods and the frustration of making and offering food to a child who rejects it. Possible solutions:

- Eat together and share only one food or only part of what your child eats.
- Make basic low-calorie foods but add calories to your child's food with extra fat or supplements.
- Join a support group with others with the same dilemma and share ideas.

Despite the challenges, if you care about what your child eats, being social and eating together is worth doing. At all ages, kids tend to eat more nutritious foods when they eat with adults. And, as kids grow older, they are more likely to eat with their parents if that pattern is established early.

INCLUDE MELLOW-OUT TIME

Before-meal activities have a way of spilling over into mealtimes. This can be especially important for a child who not only refuses to eat but also is generally defiant and uncooperative. Paying attention to the "before" mealtime can improve both the mealtime mood and a child's eating. Just before a meal, try doing something that promotes good interactions with your child.

Buzzing around with hectic activities can cause a child to be too revved up to eat. Scheduling quiet activities like setting the table or reading a book before meals helps bring down the energy level so that children are more settled and ready for eating.

OFFER EASY-TO-EAT FOODS

Choose foods that match your child's feeding skill and interest. Long before they are truly able to, kids want to feed themselves. Foods that stick to spoons and fingers make those first attempts less messy and more likely to land inside a child's mouth.

A toddler who is clumsy using utensils won't eat as much food using a fork or spoon. Finger foods are easier, less messy, and more satisfying. Most toddlers prefer foods they can pick up with their fingers. If they are sensitive to having sticky fingers, they may avoid foods that are tacky and eat only those that are dry.

Dips and sprinkles are popular with older kids and can motivate children to eat foods they would otherwise refuse. Shaking cheese onto pasta adds protein and calcium. Dunking veggies into a hummus dip adds protein, calcium, and fiber. Sprinkling wheat germ onto oatmeal adds an even longer list of nutrients.

HAVE FUN

Kids love to have fun. Use this. Build up interest in food by making up stories or names. "Munching crunchy crackers" or "Chomping chewy raisins" sounds like more fun than "Eating a snack."

You can spark interest and create anticipation for upcoming meals by talking about the foods to be eaten. Show enthusiasm whenever you eat foods that you enjoy. For young children especially, enthusiasm is contagious.

KIDS CAN HELP

two-year-olds: scrub, tear, break, snap, dip
three-year-olds: wrap, pour, mix, shake, spread
four-year-olds: peel, mash, roll, crack eggs
five-year-olds: measure, cut, grind, juice

Young children can help in the kitchen. They can open packages, and set and wipe off the table. The more involved children are with food, the more likely they are to eat.

TRY REVERSE PSYCHOLOGY

During a stage when children are playful and contrary, reverse psychology sometimes works. One clever mother noticed her son drinking less and less milk. She suspected he might drink more milk if she pretended that she did not approve. Whenever he asked for milk, she would playfully groan, "Oh, no, milk again. You want milk again. If you keep this up, I will need to buy a cow."

Another mother, whose son had medical problems that greatly complicated feeding, was determined to have him eat like everyone else. To make him want to eat, she sat him away from the table at mealtimes. As she expected, he fussed at this, demanding to be at the table. Once he was there, he went along with eating.

PRACTICE PATIENCE

Finally, parents who follow all the rules perfectly may still have a child who refuses to eat. Although there are exceptions, the general recommendation is to persevere. Hunger often drives a child to eat. Holding firm can help a child to recognize the subtle sensations of hunger rather than the social reactions their food refusals elicit. Ask your pediatrician for advice. One mother, a nurse who had a child with medically-based feeding problems, found that her child could go for days refusing food. Daily talks with the medical director of a feeding clinic gave this mother the reassurance she needed.

Neatness and Manners

Young children are messy, playful, demanding, and easily bored with food. They are bad company for adults who hope to relax and savor each bite of food or for those with high expectations for neatness and manners.

Messiness is part of the process in learning to eat independently. "Feeding the floor" is a good description for this stage. But you can help a child learn to develop better skills through play. Give a baby an empty cup to play with. Let a child practice using spoons and forks by pretending to feed dolls or puppets, or by stirring some make-believe foods in a bowl. Find nonfood ways to make messes. Being messy is not only fun for children but has benefits for sensory stimulation.

Eventually, children need to learn neatness and manners. The questions are really when and how. The one-year-old who gleefully turns his cup upside down requires a different response than a four-year-old who does the same thing. The one-year-old is engaged in discovery, while the four-year-old is demonstrating defiance. As your child grows from one stage to the next, expect fundamental changes in how he reacts to the world around him, especially food.

Match rules and expectations for mealtime behavior to your child's developmental ability. End mealtimes for one- to two-year-olds when they finish eating. Let them out of the chair, but keep them close to the table with toys on the floor. As children grow older and have longer attention spans, more language, and better social skills, encourage them to sit at the table until everyone is finished. This change comes slowly, and parents need energy, commitment, and a realistic sense of their child's skills to make it work.

Attitude

Most of the ideas in this chapter are child-focused, reflecting educational and developmental issues. While it is important to present food to children on their level, there's more to think about.

How parents approach and present food to children demonstrates their own values and attitudes. Some of these values are worth passing on while others are not. Parents with unresolved eating issues might find that thinking about their own childhood food experiences provides insights for themselves as well as for their children.

While we want eating to be enjoyable, we also need to convey the ideas that food helps our bodies grow healthy and strong and is an important part of life. There is something to be said about conveying a sense of the sacredness of what we eat and put into our bodies. Food is not a toy. In the end, eating is a serious task, necessary for good health and survival.

PART

III

Food Allergies and Digestion Problems

Your child bites into an apple, and digestion begins. Hours or days later, it ends, when what remains of the apple exits her body. In the interim, the apple undergoes an unrelenting breakdown to release nutrients. If there's a glitch somewhere along the digestive process, she might associate eating with discomfort, and, as a result, refuse to eat.

The glitch may be obvious: vomiting after eating the apple. Or it may be subtle: a burning in her throat after swallowing or a distended belly from gas or constipation. Either way, a one-time or occasional digestive glitch rarely causes a long-term food reaction. But an ongoing problem that makes a child uncomfortable will ultimately dampen her desire to eat.

This chapter looks at potential physical complications that can turn kids off to food. Regardless of whether it's aversion, allergies, constipation, or other digestive problems, parents will find ideas to help.

Aversions

One bad food experience sometimes leads to a lifelong aversion. Three-year-old Ariana once choked on a piece of celery during preschool snack. Five years later, when she sees celery, Ariana feels a lump in her throat. She can't imagine eating celery again—ever.

A traumatic food experience is hard to forget. For Ariana, the memory lingers in the body as well as the mind and includes a visceral dimension: the sight or smell alone of the offending food evokes nausea. Aversions run deeper than the typical picky-eater food refusals; they start with an unpleasant or traumatic experience.

Food aversions vary. Some, like Ariana's, are specific to one food, and others are general. Single-food aversions in older children and adults tend to be long-lasting. Broad-based aversions are common among young children who have had unpleasant oral experiences. In extreme cases, these aversions extend beyond food and include anything coming into the mouth.

While it's possible to imagine a food taste so vile as to cause an aversion, this rarely happens. A more common scenario, especially in young children, is that a food texture is too much to handle and the child chokes or vomits. Even so, a single episode rarely causes a food aversion in babies or toddlers. This changes as kids grow older. Older children or adults often tell stories of a single episode of vomiting that led to a food aversion that lasted for years.

Young children are often sensitive to food textures, and this can limit the foods they eat. Although this tendency is somewhat normal and age-related, there is a point beyond which it is called an oral aversion.

✕ *Sensory or motor-based problems often underlie food aversions. Young children are likely to have aversions to food textures rather than to specific foods. This is a sign of a sensory or motor-based problem. Chapter 8, "Food Textures and Flavors," describes activities that help kids enjoy a greater variety of food textures.*

SOCIAL INFLUENCES

There's a social as well as a biological dimension to food aversions. Younger children, at times, are surprisingly impressionable. For some, an adult's negative reaction to food, whether through word or gesture, is contagious.

The smell of hard-boiled eggs makes Josh gag. Yet Josh has never eaten a hard-boiled egg. But his father has the same reaction. Is it in their genes? Perhaps. But I suspect that Josh learned to dislike hard-boiled eggs from observing his father.

I caution adults who care for children against expressing disgust toward vegetables or other wholesome foods. In classroom observations of preschoolers, I often witness kids refusing to eat food following a single derogatory remark or facial expression.

Our social environment does influence which foods we relish and which ones we disdain. Most Americans have an aversion to eating insects. Award-winning photographer Peter Menzel proves this is not universal. He has filled a book, *Man Eating Bugs,* with images of people from around the globe eating insects with gusto.

Refusing to eat a single food, regardless of whether it is bugs or broccoli, isn't a big problem. It's the broad-based food aversions that prevent kids from eating well. These aversions are often seen in kids who have a medical history involving unpleasant experiences in the mouth.

Among the kids I work with, tube feedings are by far the most common cause. For more information on aversions in children with feeding tubes, see chapter 12, "Feeding a Child with Special Needs."

As the number of children with broad-based food aversions

grows, the therapies to treat them will continue to evolve. Nonetheless, aversions run deeper than the typical picky-eater food refusals. Don't expect to find quick or easy solutions.

Allergies

Peanut allergies are too serious and threatening to ignore. They are the leading cause of fatal and near-fatal food allergic reactions in the United States. To keep children safe, an increasing number of preschool classrooms prohibit peanut-containing foods. And parents of children with peanut allergies are advised to read food labels, to avoid travel on airlines that serve peanut snacks, to carry medication, and to take a number of other precautions.

But not all food allergies pose serious health risks. Allergic reactions can be mild and limited to something as simple as a skin rash. Allergic reactions vary, not only in intensity and symptoms (most often affecting skin, breathing, or intestines), but also in the time it takes for the reaction to occur and even the duration of the allergy. It's common for young children to outgrow their allergies. Up to 85 percent of babies who are allergic to eggs or milk outgrow their allergies by age five.

Strictly speaking, a food allergy triggers the body's immune system. Normally the immune system helps us fight off germs and disease. This powerful and protective defense system helps us resist threats from a host of threatening organisms. Yet, it is not perfect. Sometimes the body's defensive reactions are mistakenly triggered by something nonthreatening, such as food. When the trigger food is eaten, the body responds by releasing chemicals and histamines, causing the symptoms of an allergic reaction.

But there are other adverse reactions to food, which are sometimes confused with allergies. These include:

Food intolerance is not really an allergy, but rather a "side effect" reaction to the chemicals in food. Adverse effects (for example, a headache) occur after eating the food, but they are not triggered by the body's immune response. Many people have an intolerance to lactose, a sugar found in milk.

Food toxicity (poisoning) is a nonimmune reaction caused by something in food, usually bacteria or a naturally occurring substance, like caffeine.

Metabolic food reaction is a rare condition that interferes with how food chemically breaks down inside the body. An example is PKU (phenylketonuria). This genetic condition causes complications in how chemicals are processed inside the body as a result of an abnormal build up of phenylalanine, a protein building block that most people are able to process.

Because the term food allergy is often used generally to describe any adverse food reactions, some prefer to use another term—food hypersensitivity—when referring to an immune reaction to a food or a food additive.

Even though the number of young children with food allergies has risen, the overall numbers remain small, with only 2 to 8 percent of children under the age of three affected.

✕ *If you or anyone in your family has allergies, be alert. Because allergies run in families, your child will be at greater risk. If both parents have allergies, there's a 75 percent chance that their child will develop allergies. If only one parent or relative on one side of the family has allergies, there's a 30 to 40 percent chance. If neither parent has allergies, the chance is 10 to 15 percent.*

The kids most likely to be fussy eaters are those who suffer intestinal reactions soon after eating a problem food. Intestinal reactions include vomiting, nausea, stomach cramps, indigestion, and diarrhea.

It's not only physical reactions that complicate eating. There are also emotional and psychological issues for both parents and kids. When a baby is diagnosed with food allergies, parents are faced with an unexpected responsibility: learning how to handle and avoid risk foods. Meanwhile, the allergic child learns to eat more cautiously and slowly, which sometimes leads to delayed feeding skills.

As kids with allergies grow older, they worry that food may be an enemy. Suddenly social situations that involve food—school activities, birthday parties, group lunches, eating out—are less fun. It's hard to eat well when eating is stressful.

Don't make food any more of a hassle than it needs to be. Follow these basic guidelines to help your child cope with the challenges of living with food allergies:

LEARN MORE ABOUT PROBLEM FOODS

The top five foods most likely to trigger an allergic reaction in kids are milk, eggs, peanuts, wheat, and soy. Allergic reactions to milk, eggs, and peanuts account for 80 percent of all food allergies in kids under the age of three.

Milk

Millions of older kids have lactose intolerance. Although at times embarrassing and often uncomfortable, the key symptoms of lactose intolerance, gas and diarrhea, are rarely life-threatening. (For more information on this, read the section on diarrhea on page 232.)

Less common but more serious is an allergy to casein, a milk protein. If your child has an allergy to casein, you need to be more cautious. (Food allergies are potentially more serious than intolerances.) Have a plan for getting your child immediate medical care just in case someone unknowingly gives your child milk.

For children with a strong family history of allergies, it's best to delay the introduction of dairy products to one year. This includes all foods made from milk, including pudding, cheese, ice cream, and yogurt.

✕ *When naming foods that trigger an allergic reaction, choose your words carefully. When adults offer kids "milk," it is normally cow's milk. If that's not appropriate for your child, it is never too early to take precautions. Don't use the word* milk *as a generic term. Instead use the word* formula *and teach your child to drink only from a special cup. Such precautions could prevent an accident when your child is under someone else's care.*

Eggs

Eggs are an ingredient in many baked goods, especially cakes, cookies, and muffins. They are also found in custards, salad dressings, sauces, processed meats, and breading on vegetables, meats, fish, and chicken. Too often, avoiding eggs means avoiding a long list of common foods.

You can buy specialty products or learn how to modify recipes at home using substitutes. Be sure to read the labels on commercial egg substitutes carefully; some are designed to omit cholesterol and may contain egg whites.

To replace eggs in home recipes, try any of the following,

suggested by the Food Allergy and Anaphylaxis Network (each recipe equals one egg):

- 1 tsp. baking powder, 1 tbsp. liquid compatible with the recipe, and 1 tbsp. vinegar
- 1 tsp. yeast dissolved in ¼ cup warm water
- 1 tbsp. apricot puree
- 1½ tbsp. water, 1½ tbsp. oil, and 1 tsp. baking powder

Keep in mind that baking is a science and that these substitutes won't work equally well in all recipes.

For children with a strong family history of allergies, it's best to delay the introduction of eggs until age two. This includes all foods made with eggs.

Peanuts

Kids who have an allergy to peanuts are not as likely to outgrow it. They may also be allergic to other nuts. Since this allergy is long-lasting and potentially serious, parents may want to read more about the basics. One good guide is *The Peanut Allergy Answer Book,* which was written by Michael C. Yong, an allergist.

Some believe that restricting peanuts in a young child can prevent the allergy. According to the American Academy of Pediatrics, there's no guarantee that this will work, yet restriction is a sensible precaution. For children with a strong family history of allergies, delay the introduction of peanuts until they are three years old, and mothers should avoid eating peanuts during pregnancy and while breast-feeding.

✕ *Take precautions if your child has a peanut allergy. Don't take a peanut allergy lightly. Peanut allergy is the leading cause of fatal and near-fatal food allergic reactions in the United States. Plan ahead and discuss an emergency plan with your doctor.*

Wheat

Because wheat is found in so many foods, it can be difficult to avoid. Most breads, muffins, cookies, and pasta contain wheat. Small amounts are also found in sauces, soups, and breaded and processed meats. Using gluten-free foods is one way to simplify reading food labels. But a gluten-free diet is actually more restrictive than a wheat-free diet. Clarify which one your child needs.

On a wheat-free diet, foods made with the following are allowed: amaranth, arrowroot, barley, buckwheat, corn, oats, potato, quinoa, rice, rye, soybean, and tapioca. Look for these grains and foods in grocery stores, health-food stores, and mail-order catalogs. Since wheat flour is normally fortified with niacin, riboflavin, thiamine, and iron, a child on a wheat-free diet may need a supplement.

For children with a family history of allergies, it may be prudent to delay the introduction of wheat until the first birthday.

Soy

Soybeans, like peanuts, are legumes. But being allergic to more than one legume is rare. An allergy to soybeans does not necessarily mean that peanuts need to be restricted.

However, anything made with soybeans, soybean flour, or soybean protein needs to be avoided. This includes tofu, soybeans, soy grits, soy flour, soy formulas, soy granules, soy milk, soy/shoyu sauce, miso, tamari, tempeh, and textured vegetable protein (TVP). In addition, the following vaguely defined ingredients *may* contain soy or soybeans:

hydrolyzed plant protein
hydrolyzed vegetable protein
natural flavoring
vegetable broth, gums, or starch

These ingredients are found in a surprisingly large number of processed foods, which means that to avoid soy completely, you'll need to read the labels on the following products:

baked goods	cheese substitutes	milk/cream substitutes
candies	coffee replacements	meat and meat substitutes
cereals	desserts	sauces/toppings/soups

READ FOOD LABELS

Due to new regulations, reading food labels is becoming easier. As of January 1, 2006, the Food Allergen Labeling and Consumer Protection Act (FALCPA) went into effect, requiring food manufacturers to clearly list ingredients that can cause allergic reactions. The regulations apply to the eight foods that account for 90 percent of all food allergies in the United States. These foods are milk, egg, fish, crustacean shellfish, tree nuts, wheat, peanuts, and soybeans.

Before the FALCPA regulations, foods that contained milk (or a protein derived from milk) might be listed as casein or whey. For the next year or so, you may still find products on store shelves with such listings.

Because of FALCPA, the labels on any packaged foods sold in the United States must declare the presence of any of the eight foods covered in plain English. That means you will either see these foods listed in the ingredients (in understandable language) or you will see them listed in a statement that begins with "contains." In addition, foods made with nuts or seafood must list the specific type of nut or species of fish.

ALLERGY SMART
How to Read a Label

For a **milk-free** diet, avoid foods with these ingredients:

artificial butter flavor
butter, butter fat, butter
   oil
buttermilk
casein
caseinates (ammonium,
   calcium, magnesium,
   potassium, sodium)
cheese
cottage cheese
cream
curds
custard
ghee
half-and-half
hydrolysates (casein, milk
   protein, whey, whey
   protein)

lactalbumin, lactalbumin
   phosphate
lactoglobulin, lactose,
   lactulose
milk (all forms)
nougat
pudding
rennet casein
sour cream/sour milk
whey (all forms including sweet,
   delactosed, protein
   concentrate)
- "D" on a label next to "K"
   or "U" indicates presence
   of milk protein

For an **egg-free** diet, avoid foods with these ingredients:

albumin
egg (white, yolk,
   dried, powdered,
   solids)
egg substitutes
eggnog
globulin
lecithin
levetin

lysozyme (used in Europe)
mayonnaise
meringue
ovalbumin
ovomucin
ovomucoid
ovovitellin
Simplesse

(continued)

For a **peanut-free** *diet, avoid foods with these ingredients:*

beer nuts	Nu-Nuts® flavored nuts
cold-pressed peanut	peanut
oil	peanut butter
ground nuts	peanut flour
mixed nuts	

Foods that may contain peanut proteins include:

African, Chinese,	egg rolls
Indonesian, Thai, and	hydrolyzed plant protein
Vietnamese dishes	hydrolyzed vegetable protein
baked goods	marzipan
candy	nougat
chili	
chocolate	

Reprinted with permission from the Food Allergy and Anaphylaxis Network.

To make reading food labels easier, the Food Allergy and Anaphylaxis Network offers small file cards that fit into wallets or handbags and cover the common food allergies: milk, peanuts, tree nuts, soy, eggs, wheat, and shellfish.

KNOW THE SEVERITY OF YOUR CHILD'S FOOD SENSITIVITY

Kids can outgrow allergies, especially those to milk and eggs. It's a good idea to have your child retested, usually around age five, the time most kids start school. With medical documentation, public schools provide services to ensure that a child with allergies is safe. Parents need to provide EpiPens and be involved with the school to establish individualized plans for their child.

✕ *Kids with severe allergic reactions need to carry an epinephrine pen. Doctors prescribe EpiPens for kids who experience anaphy-*

laxis. Parents and caregivers can practice with a tester or with an expired "pen." Keep the EpiPens effective by storing them properly. Keep them out of sunlight and do not store in the refrigerator.

WATCH GROWTH

Kids with multiple food allergies have fewer food choices, and this makes it harder to meet nutrition needs. A study of children with food allergies found that those with two or more allergies did not grow as tall as those with only one allergy.

If your child has multiple food allergies, keep a close watch on growth. If weight or height growth drops off, consider using specialty foods or supplements to fill in nutrition gaps.

✕ *Learn to read growth charts. Keep track of your child's weight and height by plotting these on standardized growth charts (available online at www.cdc.gov). See chapter 2, "Understanding Growth," for more details.*

DON'T LET FOOD FEARS COMPLICATE LEARNING HOW TO EAT

When kids have multiple food allergies, parents are understandably more cautious about introducing new foods. But there is such a thing as being too cautious, especially with the introduction of solid foods.

Renata breast-fed her first baby and looked forward to doing so again with Alex. But after months of colic, sleepless nights, diarrhea, and poor weight gain, Alex was diagnosed as having severe food allergies. After Alex switched to a special formula he began gaining weight and life became easier.

But when Alex was six months old and ready to begin to eat solid foods, Renata was nervous. She slowly introduced pureed baby foods and avoided everything else—including dry cereal, crackers, and table foods. At sixteen months, an age at which most kids eat table foods, Alex still ate only pureed foods and turned his nose up at any food that required biting or chewing.

Despite his allergies, Alex had no problem with biting and chewing, other than a lack of experience. Learning to eat table foods was harder at sixteen months. But with patience, and help from a feeding specialist, Alex and his mom moved on to table foods.

✕ *Seek help when needed. Early Intervention is a federal entitlement program for young children. Although services vary from state to state, parents can get help for kids who have developmental delays or medical risks. A child with a delay in eating skills may be eligible for services.*

EXPAND FOOD OPTIONS—EXPERIMENT WITH COOKING

If your child is allergic to wheat, milk, or eggs, it will be hard to find appropriate breads, cookies, crackers, or cereals in your local supermarket. A health-food store will offer more choices, as will mail-order companies, such as Miss Roben's (also available on-line at www.missroben.com). Although the number of specialty products is growing, parents often feel the choices are limited and expensive.

With effort and information about nontraditional ingredients, you can make allergy-free foods at home. Start with foods that freeze easily. If they are not a hit the first time, you can try again. You'll need a specialized cookbook, such as

The Allergy Self-Help Cookbook (**2nd edition**) by Marjorie Hurt Jones. Rodale Press, 2001.

This 416-page book is filled with recipes free of wheat, milk, egg, corn, and other common food allergens.

The Food Allergy News Cookbook by the Food Allergy and
Anaphylaxis Network. John Wiley & Sons, 1998.
In addition to recipes coded for food allergies (milk, eggs,
peanuts, wheat, soy, and nuts), there are tips on preparing allergy-free foods and useful substitutions.

Special Foods for Special Kids by Todd Adelman and Jodi
Behrend. Reed Publishers, 1999.
This book features one hundred "child-approved" recipes that
are categorized by meal. Each recipe includes nutrient analysis
and substitutions to make foods dairy-, egg-, or wheat-free.

HELP YOUR CHILD COPE

Kids with food restrictions often feel left out. Prepare your
child in advance for treat-oriented holidays, like Halloween, and
for social situations where food is a focus. To talk to your child
about both feelings and food safety, the following resources can
help:

Alexander **series.** Food Allergy Network, 1999.
This series of food-allergy books helps elementary-school
children better understand and cope with food restrictions.
There is also a video about Alexander, the elephant who can't
eat peanuts.

The Peanut Butter Jam by Elizabeth Sussman Nassau. Health
Press, 2001.
This book, for ages four to eight, tells the story of a peanut-
allergic boy who feels left out when his classmates make
peanut butter birdfeeders. It explains an anaphylactic reaction
to peanuts and what needs to be done.

Taking Food Allergies to School by Ellen Weiner. JayJo Books, 1999.

This book talks about common food situations that kids encounter in school: sharing lunches, attending parties, and buying snacks. It includes tips for teachers.

A basic problem that all parents confront is that when kids don't feel well, they don't eat well. Congestion and problems with breathing make it harder to eat and harder to enjoy food. Any allergy, even a nonfood one, can cause the appetite to drop.

Alexandra had mild allergies to pollen. So in late spring when the pollen count was high, she was sniffly and congested. At eighteen months, her eating was not great, and she had a history of vomiting. Congestion didn't help. In the spring, everything got worse.

One spring morning Alexandra's mother ignored the kitchen mess and focused her attention on her daughter. As she watched Alexandra nibble on toast, she wondered: Could the extra mucus in her daughter's nose and throat make eating uncomfortable? Later she called the doctor, who agreed that the mucus could complicate Alexandra's ability to coordinate eating and breathing. He suggested giving Alexandra a saline nasal spray before meals. The simple solution helped, as Alexandra ate more and vomited less.

✕ *Over-the-counter decongestants have side effects. A saline spray (basically salty sterile water) is relatively benign. Other over-the-counter decongestants are more likely to have side effects. Antihistamines often cause drowsiness and oral decongestants can interfere with sleep, appetite, and mood.*

Constipation

Constipation isn't glamorous, but it is common. Among the young children I see, constipation is a routine complaint, and even a mild case affects a small child's appetite. Two-year-old Kiara is one of the picky eaters I have followed for more than a year. On most days, Kiara has a bowel movement. But on the days that she does not, her mother has noticed that Kiara eats less.

What is constipation? Comparing how often one child has bowel movements to another doesn't offer clear answers. Some kids go only once every three or four days while others go several times a day. At the very least, a child (or adult) needs to defecate at least once a week. Babies may have a bowel movement after every feeding, but as they grow older and bigger, things slow down. By age three, children average one to two bowel movements a day. After age four, children pass the same number of stools a day as adults do.

If you suspect that your child is constipated, look for these signs:

- Painful bowel movements
- Hard stools, especially if they are small and pelletlike
- Bleeding or severe straining are clear signs of a problem.
- Less clear is a child who looks uncomfortable. Babies often make faces, but toddlers and preschoolers tend to hide while going.

If your child suffers from constipation, try making simple food changes as the first step toward a solution. Usually that means increasing fiber and fluids, and sometimes decreasing milk. As a start, try these ideas:

DOES YOUR CHILD NEED MORE FLUIDS?

Check your child's urine pattern.

- Kids in diapers should wet four or five diapers a day.
- Toilet-trained kids typically urinate at least once every five or six hours.

INCREASE WATER

Water dilutes food contents in the GI tract and helps move everything through and out. Encourage your child to drink more water. If she refuses plain water, try diluting it with fruit juice. Prune juice is the best laxative. If that doesn't work, try pear nectar.

Keep in mind that many solid foods are also high in fluids. Most fruits and many vegetables are high in fluids, as are Popsicles and gelatin.

INCREASE ACTIVITY

Encourage your child to move. Movement of the lower body through walking or crawling stimulates the muscles in the large intestine and can promote bowel movements. For babies, massage has a similar effect.

HOW MUCH FIBER DO KIDS NEED?

Age	Grams of fiber per day
2	7
3	8
4	9
5	10

FINDING FIBER-RICH FOODS

Food	Amount	Grams of Fiber
Baked beans	½ cup	9
Kidney beans	½ cup	7
Navy beans	½ cup	6
Lima beans	½ cup	5
Sweet potato	1 medium	4
Peas	¼ cup	4
Tomato (raw)	1 large	4
Apple	1 medium	3
Pear	½ large	3
Raisins	3 tbsp.	3
Broccoli	½ cup	2
Carrots, boiled	½ cup	2
Dates	3	2
Peach	1 medium	2
Prunes	2 medium	2
Grapes	1 cup	1

INCREASE FIBER

Even kids need fiber. The recommended amount increases as they grow older. See the chart below. (The amount of fiber recommended for children under the age of two is not yet established.) The maximum amount of fiber recommended for adolescents is twenty grams.

Encouraging kids to eat plant-based foods will increase fiber intake, but the amounts vary greatly from one fruit or vegetable to another. Use the chart on the following page as a general guide.

Increase fiber by using high-fiber breads and cereals. Look

for the Dietary Fiber listing on the Nutrition Facts panel. Whole-grain breads generally provide up to three grams of fiber per slice; cereals vary. The chart below lists the fiber content of some ready-to-eat cereals. If the high-fiber cereals are not a hit, try mixing them in with a cereal your child normally eats.

FIBER IN READY-TO-EAT CEREALS	
Cereal	*Fiber in ½-cup serving*
Bran Buds	18
All-Bran with extra fiber	15.5
Fiber One	13
All-Bran	10
Wheat germ	7
Grape-Nuts	5
Cracklin' Oat Bran	4
Multi-Bran Chex	3.5
Raisin Bran	3.5
Mini-Wheats	3
Fruit & Fibre	2.5
Shredded Wheat	2.5
Wheat Chex	2.5

LIMIT LOW-FIBER AND CONSTIPATING FOODS

When kids fill up on milk, yogurt, white bread, meat, and maca-roni and cheese, they are more likely to be constipated. These low-fiber foods don't provide much roughage, which helps move everything into the large bowel and out.

If your child drinks more than twenty-four ounces of milk a day and likes cheese and other dairy foods, try cutting the milk down to sixteen ounces a day. This will make your child hungrier and more likely to eat high-fiber foods.

TRY POOP GOOP

If simple food changes don't work and you want to try something more powerful without using a stool softener, you can try a recipe I like to call Poop Goop.

Or buy Fruit-Eze, which is a fruit paste made from prunes, dates, and raisins. It doesn't need refrigeration and has a shelf life of one year after opening. Order it online from www.fruit-eze.com or call 1-888-regular.

You can also order high-fiber cookies (with three to five grams of fiber per cookie) or high-fiber juice (with ten grams of fiber per eight-ounce juice box) from www.nutra-balance-products.com (800-432-3134) or Lori's Earth Friendly Products www.earth-friendly.com (732-937-5978). Some of these require a bulk purchase.

POOP GOOP I	**POOP GOOP II**
1 cup raisins	1 orange
1 cup prunes	1 apple (with skin)
¼ cup dates	1 cup raisins
8 ounces prune juice	1 cup prunes
	½ cup prune juice
	½ cup orange juice
Mix together in a blender or food processor. Store in the refrigerator. Use 1–2 table-spoons per day.	Mix together in a blender or food processor. Store in the refrigerator. Use 1–2 table-spoons per day.

CONSTIPATION AND TOILET TRAINING

The transition from diapers can be stressful. During toilet training, some kids withhold bowel movements. Parents can help by trying to decrease a child's fears and by increasing fiber and fluids. If these simple measures don't work, get medical advice.

If your child is at this stage, in addition to food changes, help your child establish regular bowel habits:

- Set aside a quiet, unrushed time for toileting. At the same time each day, put your child on the toilet. Try to do it within thirty minutes after a meal, since eating or drinking often stimulates intestinal activity.
- Encourage your child to sit for several minutes. If he needs motivation to sit, offer stickers or other age-appropriate rewards.
- Try to maintain an easygoing attitude about your child's toileting. If he is anxious or afraid, you'll need to be reassuring.

✕ *Use a story to make bowel movements less frightening. Reading a picture book such as* Everyone Poops *by Taro Gomi, telling stories, or simply talking it through can help make your child more comfortable with this new experience.*

IF CONSTIPATION DOESN'T GO AWAY . . .

Poor appetite and poor school performance are not the only the symptoms associated with constipation. For some children the symptoms are more severe.

Five-year-old Tom never had a problem until he started school. He did not like using the bathroom at school and waited until he went home to use the toilet. As a result, he began to withhold his stool voluntarily. After a while, this caused a large mass of stool to accumulate in his rectum. The mass got dried out, becoming harder to pass. Eventually his rectal muscles became fatigued and small amounts of fecal material from high in the colon leaked through (the medical term for this is fecal soiling or encopresis). Tom had no sensation or control over this. Because Tom was potty-trained, his parents didn't immediately recognize that he was having a problem.

In order to defecate we need to relax. Passing stools requires a combination of learned and involuntary behaviors. Feces eventually collects in the lowest part of the bowel, the rectum. Two muscles prevent the feces from leaking out: the internal anal sphincter and the external anal sphincter. We control defecation by squeezing the external muscle. But we have no control over the internal muscles, which reflexively relax when stool enters the rectum. When the stool enters the rectum it presses on the external sphincter, creating the urge to defecate. If both muscles relax, the stool passes out of the body. If the muscles don't relax or one contracts the external sphincter, the stool moves back up into the colon and the urge to defecate goes away.

While the mechanism of how this happens is straightforward, the causes are not. There are a number of less common biological conditions that can lead to constipation. These range from pain caused by a crack or fissure in the anus (a very common problem in children) to anorectal trauma to neurological conditions (spina bifida, sacral agenesis, pelvic trauma, diseases causing hypotonia, or motor incoordination). Anything that causes dehydration (from gastroenteritis, vomiting, malnutrition, or diabetes) is also a possible cause. Constipation can also be a side effect of taking certain drugs (including diuretics and antihistamines).

To help a child with constipation, increase fiber, fluids, and movement. But be prepared to use stool softeners or laxatives. Jonah had a long-standing problem with constipation, and extra fiber and fluids were not enough to help him. The gastroenterologist who treated him put him on a stool softener and recommended keeping him on it for several months. Because having bowel movements was painful for Jonah, he was not able to relax. Instead, when he felt an urge to move his bowels, he withheld to avoid pain. The doctor suggested that using the stool softener for four months would help him to disassociate pain with passing a stool.

A child who has had long-term constipation may have tried any number of products. But not all laxatives work the same way. The mild ones (such as psyllium) are bulk-forming and work the same way as fiber in food. As they pass through the digestive system they absorb water, and the soft bulky mass helps to push things through. For some, it is critical to use extra fluids; otherwise the constipation may worsen.

Another class of laxatives is known as emollients. Mineral oil is one of these. As indigestible fat, it passes into the large intestine, making the undigested food mass more slippery. Eventually the food mass slides through.

The most heavy-duty class of laxatives (such as those containing senna) work on the central nervous system. It sends messages to the muscles in the large intestine to contract, and, as a result, feces are pushed out. While powerful, these laxatives are the most likely to become habit-forming.

BEYOND FOOD

The following is a partial list of laxatives and stool softeners. For children under the age of three, it's best to be cautious. Talk to your doctor before using any laxative.

NONPRESCRIPTION
Benefiber
This tasteless, odorless powder can be added to drinks.

Malt Supex

This is often used with infants and young children, but a bottle can cost more than forty dollars. For children older than one, barley malt, available in health-food stores, is cheaper but less convenient to mix.

Metamucil (Psyllium)

This bulk fiber needs to be given with plenty of water. It can also be used in recipes with gelatin.

Mineral Oil

This is an old-fashioned emollient that makes stools soft and slippery. However, it can interfere with the absorption of some nutrients.

Milk of Magnesia

This is a saline laxative that works by drawing water into the stool. Small dosages are sometimes used with children over the age of two. High doses of magnesium can be toxic for children, so don't use this without a physician's approval.

PRESCRIPTION

Your child's doctor will choose one based on experience and your child's needs. Examples of medications that might be recommended include **Colace, lactulose, MiraLax, and Senokot.**

In general, it's best to start with simple solutions, such as dietary changes, to solve a child's constipation. But if the problem persists, don't hesitate to seek medical advice. For some children, constipation is difficult to treat. In fact, it is the second most common reason why pediatricians refer children to a gastrointestinal specialist.

DEHYDRATION—WHO IS AT RISK?

Kids under the age of two or kids who weigh less than twenty-five pounds.

Replacing fluids—what's best?

Commercial products like Pedialyte. Soft drinks and juice, although better when diluted with water, are not as effective and in some instances can actually increase the risk of dehydration.

The problem—will kids drink it?

Sometimes kids refuse to drink the rehydration fluid because of the salty taste. You can try using it in freeze pops or looking for a flavored one.

Diarrhea

Usually when a child has diarrhea, it is a short-term problem. During the week or two that children are sick, they may eat next to nothing. But, like the diarrhea itself, the drop in appetite is temporary.

Diarrhea often goes away on its own. But any type of diarrhea or other condition that causes a fluid loss brings a risk of dehydration.

✕ *Use oral rehydration fluids to prevent dehydration. Don't expect these special drinks to stop the diarrhea—they don't. Diarrhea often continues for three to seven days. But using these drinks does reduce the risk that your child will become dehydrated.*

When a young child has diarrhea, it's best to consult with a doctor. When you do, be prepared to answer questions about details of the diarrhea and lifestyle information on day care, travel, food, and animal contacts. In some cases, you may need to collect a stool sample.

INFECTIOUS DIARRHEA

Often, diarrhea is infectious, spreading from the outside world to your child through a virus, bacteria, or parasite. Exactly which one varies from one part of the world to another. In North America, rotavirus is common, and almost all children living in the United States experience this infection by the time they are four or five years old. Rotavirus infection causes an explosive, watery diarrhea.

Infectious diarrhea can also spread through contaminated food or water. When traveling to a foreign country with a young child, you may need to avoid the local water and limit the raw foods your child eats. Sanitation standards vary, and young children have less resistance to infections. Check out the CDC Web site, www.cdc.gov, for specific recommendations for the country in which you plan to travel.

✕ *Keep foods at home safe to eat.*
- *Scrub cutting boards with soap and water after raw poultry has been on them. Use different cutting boards for breads, salads, and other noncooked foods.*
- *Do not give your child uncooked or soft-boiled eggs. They could contain salmonella.*
- *Defrost foods in the refrigerator or microwave, not on the counter. Bacteria grow fastest at room temperature.*
- *Prevent cross-contamination by washing anything that touches raw meat, fish, or poultry.*
- *Keep dirty diapers separate from food and food-preparation areas.*
- *Wash your hands after changing diapers or handling risky foods.*

The list of potential causes of infectious diarrhea is endless and the symptoms vary with each type. With some, it is simply diarrhea, while with others there could be fever, vomiting, and cramping. Doctors generally don't give children medications for the common forms of diarrheal infections. Although these are unpleasant to live through, kids often recover without treatment.

DIARRHEA AND FOOD

Not all diarrhea comes from infections. Food sensitivities are associated with noninfectious diarrhea. In this case, there is no germ to blame, but a child's body is reacting to something in the food itself. Sometimes this is known as "toddler's diarrhea."

SORBITOL IN JUICES	
Type	*Grams per 3.3 ounces*
Prune	12.7
Pear	2.1
Sweet cherry	1.4
Peach	0.9
Apple	0.5
Grape	trace

Juice

Every day, two-year-old Carlos had four loose stools. At first, his mom thought he might have food allergies. Even though Carlos was a picky eater, he was not a picky drinker. He loved to drink apple juice and normally drank five cups a day. Once he cut back on the juice, Carlos stopped having loose stools.

Fruit juices such as apple, pear, and prune contain sorbitol, a nonabsorbable sugar that moves through a child's sensitive body, causing toddler's diarrhea.

Fat

What is good nutrition for adults is not always good for young children—especially in regard to fat. While most adults benefit from eating less fat, children do not. For toddlers, too little fat can actually cause diarrhea.

Tina had been a dancer through high school and college. She counted every gram of fat in the foods she ate. Her two-year-old daughter, Olivia, ate the same foods that she ate: lots of fruits and vegetables, lean meats, 1 percent fat milk, and no cheese. While this food combination worked well for Tina, it was a problem for Olivia, who was underweight and had very loose stools.

Toddlers need 30 to 40 percent of calories from fat. Tina's were 10 to 15 percent—this was too low for her daughter. Olivia's stools became normal after she started drinking whole milk and eating cheese.

Lactose

A third cause of noninfectious food-related diarrhea in children is lactose, a sugar found in milk. The body's ability to break down lactose is fragile and easily disrupted. For some, lactose intolerance is a temporary condition—a lingering effect following antibiotic use (as might happen with an ear infection), infectious diarrhea, or some other intestinal upset. Whatever the duration or cause, the key symptoms of lactose intolerance, namely gas and diarrhea, though at times uncomfortable, are rarely life-threatening.

✕ *Use special products to decrease lactose. You can buy ready-to-use reduced-lactose milk, such as Lactaid, or Lactaid drops that can be*

HOW MUCH LACTOSE IS IN FOODS?

Food	Grams of lactose
1 cup milk	11
½ cup half-and-half	5
1 cup lactose-reduced milk	3
1 tsp. butter/margarine	trace
½ cup cottage cheese	3
1 cup yogurt	5
1 ounce cheese	1–2
½ cup ice cream	6–9

added to regular milk to break down the lactose. You can also talk to your child's doctor about using lactase enzyme tablets, which can be taken with a meal containing lactose.

IF DIARRHEA DOESN'T GO AWAY

Long-term diarrhea often interferes with a child's growth and is therefore more serious. Diarrhea causes everything to move through the digestive system at a faster rate—usually too fast for all nutrients and calories to be absorbed.

From the beginning, three-year-old Todd was a puzzle—a small, underweight boy with a supersized appetite. He lived with his grandmother, who said, "He eats everything—he is not fussy." The food diary she kept confirmed this. Todd ate mountains of food, enough to provide 50 percent more calories than a boy his size and age normally needs to gain weight. Yet Todd was falling off the growth curve.

After seeing a specialist, Todd was diagnosed with celiac disease. Todd had persistent diarrhea—the classic symptom of celiac disease. The solution was a gluten-free diet, which meant that Todd couldn't eat anything made with wheat, rye, or barley.

In recent years, the tests for celiac disease have become more sophisticated, and experts now recognize that there are children with celiac disease who have nonclassic symptoms, which include constipation and poor appetite. New tests make screening for celiac disease easier.

Other conditions that can cause long-term diarrhea include food allergy/intolerance, medications, short-gut syndrome, and cystic fibrosis. When diarrhea lasts longer than two weeks, it becomes a threat to a child's health and nutrition. Kids suffering from long-term diarrhea may eat well but they rarely grow well. Any child with long-term diarrhea needs medical care to find the cause and, eventually, the treatment.

Reflux

The front of two-year-old Dylan's T-shirt was always wet. His parents changed it four times each day. Usually they found it hard to tell whether he had drooled, belched, or spit up.

Baby spit-up, otherwise known as reflux, is something that most kids outgrow by their first birthday or by the time they are able to stand or walk. In reflux, more accurately called gastroesophageal reflux (GER) or gastroesophageal reflux disease (GERD), the contents of the stomach travel back up into the esophagus instead of moving down into the stomach. This happens because the sphincter muscle at the top of the stomach doesn't stay closed. In babies this muscle is immature and, as a result, spitting up is common.

Even though reflux is common, sometimes the symptoms are more severe. Talk about any of the following with your child's doctor:

- **Vomiting** Report vomiting that is frequent, or contains blood or green or yellow fluid. Repeated vomiting can also cause poor weight gain.

- *Inconsolable crying and irritability* These are signs of pain. Food that is refluxed from the stomach into the esophagus contains acid, which causes a burning sensation.
- *Poor appetite and poor growth* Kids with ongoing reflux are at risk for problems with weight gain.
- *Breathing problems* When food travels back up the esophagus it sometimes starts to go into the lungs. This can interfere with breathing. Possible symptoms of this include wheezing, chronic cough, recurrent pneumonia, hoarseness, and, sometimes, asthma. In a child without a cold or flu, these are flags to see a doctor, preferably a specialist such as a gastroenterologist.

In addition to medication, there are other interventions that can help to reduce reflux. These include:

- **Upright position** Gravity helps keep the contents of the stomach from flowing up rather than down. Avoid having your child lie down after meals. At night, a wedge placed under the mattress can elevate the top of the bed.
- **Low activity level** No jumping, skipping, or running after eating. Plan quiet activities after meals. Delayed gastric emptying time is common among children with reflux, meaning that food sits in the stomach longer than usual. Vigorous activities prevent gravity from pulling food down into the intestines, where it needs to go.
- **Loose clothing** Avoid tight diapers and elastic waistbands, which can increase stomach pressure.
- **Frequent meals** Overeating stuffs too much food into the stomach. This makes it easier for it to move back up. Smaller and more frequent meals help. For children over the age of two, avoid eating two to three hours before bedtime.

- **Formula** In some cases, specialized formulas are worth a try. These include prethickened ones, for babies, or those made with whey protein, which are available for all ages. Another common remedy involves thickening formula with baby cereal. This changes the calorie and nutrient concentration of the formula (and sometimes causes constipation). Talk to a dietitian or doctor to find out if any of these might be helpful for your child.
- **Eliminate acidic foods** Because foods can trigger the stomach to release more acid and make the reflux worse, it's worthwhile to eliminate the following: carbonated drinks, chocolate, caffeine, foods that are high in fat (such as French fries and pizza), high-acid foods (such as citrus, pickles, and tomatoes), and spicy foods. Try the food changes for a few weeks. Since these changes don't always reduce reflux, continue the restrictions only if it helps.
- **Avoid tobacco smoke** Keep your child away from cigarette smoke.

Doctors often prescribe medication to treat reflux. The most common are:

- **Acid blockers** These are the medications most often used to treat reflux. They work by reducing acid production at the source—the stomach. Zantac and Prilosec are the ones most often used for children. These drugs are available over the counter for adults and kids over the age of twelve. Younger children need a prescription in order to get the correct dosage for their body size.
- **Acid neutralizers** These old-fashioned remedies are available over the counter. They include Tums, Rolaids, Maalox, Mylanta, Alka-Seltzer, and Riopan. Although occasionally

used for short-term treatment in children and adolescents, they are not recommended for long-term use. Generally, other drug treatments are considered to be more convenient and safe for use in young children.

• **Promotility agents** These work by helping food to move faster from the stomach into the small intestine. Often children with reflux have delayed gastric emptying time. A medicine such as Reglan (metoclopramide) stimulates the stomach to work faster. However, there are potential side effects, the worst of which is severe muscle spasms that can come on suddenly. Benadryl can be used to counteract this.

A newer and more effective drug, Propulsid (cisapride), was removed from the U.S. market because of safety concerns. It is sometimes available under research programs that require strict monitoring.

SOMETIMES REFLUX IS NOT REFLUX

There's another condition that has similar symptoms to reflux but is actually an allergic reaction known as eosinophil esophagitis (EE). EE is on the rise in both children and adults. In this condition, the esophagus becomes inflamed due to a type of white blood cell known as eosinophils. High levels of these eosinophils indicate an allergic reaction.

There are variations of EE, such as EG (eosinophilic gastroenteritis), where there's inflammation in the stomach and small intestine; or EC (eosinophilic colitis), where the inflammation is in the large bowel. In all versions, it is believed that the body is reacting to whole food proteins. The primary cure is to restrict the trigger foods from the diet.

The foods most likely to cause EE are cow's milk, soy, egg, and wheat. To confirm whether a child has EE or reflux, he needs to be seen by a specialist.

Vomiting

There's a surprisingly long list of conditions that cause vomiting, including any number of bacteria, viruses, allergies, toxins, physical obstructions, oral aversions, and intolerances. Although common, vomiting is potentially serious, and it is a problem you should discuss with your child's pediatrician. Any child with severe or prolonged vomiting needs to be seen by a physician.

✕ *When vomiting is prolonged or severe, give your child extra fluids. Dehydration is a serious health risk for small children. Offer sips of water, ice chips, fruit juice diluted half-and-half with water, a commercial rehydration drink like Pedialyte, or a flat soft drink. If your child is too sick to drink, call your pediatrician immediately.*

Some children vomit easily, and instead of provoking a crisis, vomiting turns into an everyday occurrence. Even then, vomiting can never be completely dismissed. A child who vomits easily often has one or more of the following:

- Oral sensitivity
- Delayed feeding skills
- Poor growth
- Allergies
- Reflux

None of these can be ignored and each one is discussed elsewhere in this book. While any complication that affects eating needs to be addressed, it's often best to make decreasing the vomiting the first priority.

Madison had delayed feeding skills. At one year she ate only stage one baby foods. Whenever she tried anything more difficult, she threw up. While the vomiting was unpleasant, her parents' greatest concern was that Madison was not yet eating table foods like other one-year-olds. They felt they needed to encourage her to eat more difficult foods, otherwise she would continue to fall further behind.

In fact, Madison made more progress after her parents shifted their focus to decreasing the vomiting. Each time it happened they noticed what triggered it and tried to avoid it. Sometimes it was food, sometimes it was being picked up too quickly or crying too long. Soon Madison's vomiting decreased from once or twice a day to once a month and it continued to drop over the next few months.

At the same time, they did oral-motor exercises recommended by a therapist and started over with more difficult solid foods. Three months later, the vomiting had stopped and Madison was eating table foods.

Madison had persistent vomiting that started at an early age and had a physical basis. But there are emotional causes as well. Stressful life changes, like a move, a divorce, a new sibling, or other family upheavals, upset kids and may cause vomiting. Sometimes kids cry so intensely that they vomit. This is especially common between the ages of eighteen months and four years, a time of increasing independence and defiance.

VOMITING AT WILL

Normally vomiting is involuntary, a reaction triggered by a variety of biological conditions. But over time, vomiting can change from an involuntary reaction to a voluntary act. Most people, including young children, can learn how to vomit at will. This is a problem, especially when a two-year-old masters the method.

An important prerequisite that enables a young child to learn how to vomit voluntarily is practice. Young children who already vomit daily are at greatest risk. Once a child reaches the stage where vomiting is voluntary, it is even harder for him to stop.

Unfortunately, kids who become practiced at this art gain attention and a sense of power. Few things get a parent's attention faster than vomiting up a good meal.

Once a child has learned to vomit at will, parents can still break the pattern, especially if it hasn't gone on too long. The first step is finding out whether or not the child has learned to control when they vomit.

Parents who repeatedly clean up after a child's vomit often tune in to early warning signs. These vary for each child. Some parents tell me that they recognize a certain look on a child's face or a change in body position. Being aware of telltale signs that occur *before* a child vomits is helpful. This is an important step in reversing the pattern.

Is vomiting intentional? Once you see a warning sign, find out by distracting your child with an unexpected noise or other quick-action surprise. Be sure the distraction occurs in the few seconds *before* your child vomits. A noise that startles rather than frightens a child works best. If the distraction stops the child from vomiting, it is a sign that it is voluntary.

The big risk is that your child will learn to use vomiting as a behavior to control you. This is less likely to happen if you can ignore your child's provocative behavior. Admittedly, this is difficult to do. There are suggestions on this in chapter 9, "Family Influences." But normally this is difficult to overcome without support. Talk to your child's pediatrician for suggestions. This problem is easier to deal with if you address it early.

Food allergies and digestive problems take many forms. Becoming more informed about the treatments will enable you to understand whether any of them are contributing to your child's picky eating.

Do

- Educate yourself about digestive conditions that may affect your child's appetite.
- Ensure your child drinks extra fluids when she vomits, has diarrhea, or a fever. Any of these increases the risk for dehydration.
- Watch what your child drinks. Too much juice is a common cause of a toddler's diarrhea.
- Discuss any problems your child has with vomiting with the pediatrician.

Don't

- Ignore constipation. There are a variety of solutions to keep your child regular.
- Thoughtlessly make negative remarks about wholesome food. Ideas can be contagious.
- Assume your child has a food allergy. Many reactions are actually food intolerances, which are less serious.

Feeding a Child with Special Needs

The number of children with special needs has risen over the last twenty-five years. Enrollment in special education preschool programs nationally grew from 360,000 in 1988 to 571,000 in 1997. This is partly because the modern definition of a special needs child is broader than it was in the past. It includes not only children with specific medical conditions but also those who need more care or support than average. To be precise, the official definition used by the Maternal and Child Health Bureau of the federal government states:

> Children who have special health care needs are those who have . . . a chronic physical, developmental, behavioral, or emotional condition and who also require health and related services of a type or amount beyond that required by children generally.

Given the broad definition, it's not surprising that special needs children are a remarkably diverse group. Despite the differences, they are likely to have one thing in common: a struggle with food. Researchers estimate that up to 80 percent of kids with special needs have feeding problems. Because eating is a complex process, a broad range of problems arise. Children with special needs may have difficulties with feeding or growth, and sometimes they need food restrictions or specialized formulas.

Who are these children? Those with autism, prematurity, cerebral palsy, Down syndrome, and other syndromes and congenital conditions often need extra help with feeding.

Feeding Challenges

The feeding challenges a child with special needs is likely to face include slow progression to table foods, rigid food preferences, and slow growth.

SLOW FOOD PROGRESSIONS

Young children, especially those with special needs, vary in their readiness to handle food-texture transitions—from liquids to pureed foods or from pureed foods to solids. While the majority of children learn to eat a full range of food textures, some do it at a slower pace. This is common among children with any of the following:

Cerebral palsy
Cornelia de Lang syndrome
Down syndrome—trisomy 21
Down syndrome—trisomy 18
Fragile X syndrome
Lowe syndrome
Marfan syndrome
Rett syndrome
Williams syndrome

Many children without a specific diagnosis or recognized medical problem have difficulty with food transitions. Generally, in order to keep meals enjoyable, parents need to wait until a child is ready for new food experiences. There are signs you can look for to recognize when your child is ready to move from one stage of eating to the next. Chapter 3, "Feeding Skills," gives basic guidelines on prerequisite skills that children need to eat different types of food.

At the same time, parents may need to prod a child forward gently. Often there's work to be done. Before they move forward, children may need to develop better postural strength, improve mouth-muscle movements, or overcome oral aversions. The tasks vary from one child to the next. It can be difficult to find the right balance between waiting for readiness and being proactive in helping the child move forward. Talking to another parent with a special needs child, a therapist, or an adult who knows your child can help.

If your child struggles with food transitions, follow the basic feeding guidelines below. These are general guidelines and may not address all of your child's needs. For that, you'll need to consult with a specialist who can watch your child eat and offer specific recommendations.

> The mother of a child with Down syndrome, who also happens to be a dietitian, has written guidelines on feeding to help other parents. In addition to practical tips, she offers insights on how to achieve a balance between waiting for a child to be ready and being more aggressive with feeding. Joan Medlen's "From Milk to Table Foods: A Parent's Guide to Introducing Food Textures" is available online at www.altonweb.com/cs/downsyndrome/index.htm. This guide contains practical advice for any parent whose child is moving slowly toward eating table foods.

BASIC FEEDING GUIDELINES FOR CHILDREN
WITH SPECIAL NEEDS

1. Find a comfortable position for you and your child. Normally, it's best to have a child sit with feet on the floor (or on a foot rest) and the head straight (rather than tilted back). Good posture helps too. Technically, that means that a child's knees, hips, and elbows are flexed at a 90-degree angle.

2. If your child needs to be fed, establish a routine that signals that food is coming or tell your child that it is time to eat. Do this regardless of whether your child is talking. Pay attention to the pace of feeding. Find a rhythm—slow, moderate, or fast—that works best for your child.

3. If your child is able to feed himself, be social and eat together. When children watch others eat, it makes it easier to learn that eating can be enjoyable.

4. Activities that focus on the mouth can help children feel more comfortable with eating. Before meals, try gently massaging the inside of your child's mouth. Use a mirror to point out tongue, lips, and teeth. Play games that encourage blowing, kissing, or yawning. Make sounds that involve exaggerated lip movements, such as "ba-ba," "boo-boo," "pop-pop."

5. Match food textures to your child's skill and comfort level. Advance textures slowly. To ensure that a child eats enough, include favorite foods along with more challenging ones.

6. When giving solid foods, remind your child to chew. Don't hesitate to model and chew with your mouth open or to simply say, "Chew, chew, chew." You can also let the child *feel* your jaw while you chew.

7. Give your child praise for chewing and trying new foods.

8. Experiment with cups, straws, and utensils to find those that make eating easier and fun.

9. If your child refuses food or spits it out, watch your own reactions. It's usually best to stay quiet or make neutral comments.

10. If your child gags, stay calm and alert. Give your child a moment to recover before you give help.

RIGID FOOD PREFERENCES

Despite parents' best efforts, there are times when a child has trouble with physical, sensory, or emotional aspects of eating. Any of these can lead a child to become rigidly resistant to new foods, leaving parents frustrated, worried about nutrition, and unsure of how to initiate changes.

Rigid eating is especially common among children who have autism. In a survey done through the Autism Project at the University of Louisville's Child Evaluation Center, the majority of parents (67 percent) described their children as picky eaters. The typical problems were "unwillingness to try new foods," "mouthing objects," and "rituals around eating."

At first, the term "unwillingness to try new foods" barely sounds worrisome. Yet when one takes a closer look at the rigid eating and other problems around food that many parents confront, it is easy to understand why they *do* worry or at least feel very frustrated. Some autistic children have delays in eating and self-feeding skills. Some simply have an extremely short and unchanging list of acceptable foods. Despite the tendency to be picky about which foods they will eat, most eat reasonable quantities of food provided they are given the foods that they like. As a consequence, they tend to grow well. In fact, many health professionals don't realize that eating is an issue because the majority of children with autism are average size or large for their age.

Children with autism are often diagnosed between the ages of two and four, which means that their parents are likely to struggle with eating problems on their own for a while. Parents may not get support or professional help until the child has a diagnosis.

Rigid food refusals are also found in children with aversions. These may be innate or acquired as a result of unpleasant experiences in the mouth or with eating. Children with aversions and autism often have strong sensory reactions to food and are prone to resist new foods, so that what are sometimes dismissed as typical toddler food jags are, in fact, much more extreme. If your child's resistance to new foods is extreme, you should not ignore it. You can help him expand the foods he will accept by paying more attention to the textures and flavors of the foods you offer. Details on this are discussed in chapter 8, "Food Textures and Flavors." In addition, feeding specialists recommend the following strategies:

Set a Consistent Mealtime Pattern

Consistency and sameness help many children eat and behave better. Predictable mealtime routines offer structure and reassurance, which are comforting. It is often worth the effort to have a consistent schedule, location, surroundings, activities, and companions. Additionally, often a child eats better if all the food interactions take place with the same person.

When a child attends school or day care, coordinate the schedule and structure to ensure that there's consistency between meals that take place inside and outside the home.

Redefine Eating

At times, children are so resistant to new foods that even the presence of an unacceptable food on the table or plate is upsetting. For example, if Jacob's mother puts turkey on his plate, he won't eat *anything* until she removes the offensive turkey. In such instances, *any* step toward accepting food is progress, even when the food is not eaten.

Kay Toomey, a feeding specialist, has outlined a "Steps to Eating" guide based on the idea that eating is a multistep process that for some children begins with accepting the presence of new foods. This approach takes the child's starting point into account and breaks down the process of accepting foods into small incremental steps. Allowing food on the table or plate and touching or smelling foods are all steps toward acceptance. Eventually children progress to licking, biting, and actually swallowing new foods. Unfortunately, this can be a slow process that takes months. Nonetheless, it's important to reward *any* interaction that a child has with food and recognize that it is progress.

Minimize Stimuli or Distractions

When children are on the edge of being able to focus on food, it doesn't take much to distract them from eating. A simple solution is to minimize distractions during meals.

Some children have strong reactions to outside stimulation. The distractions may be obvious, such as loud noise, too many people, or too much commotion. Yet when children are sensitive, distractions may be subtle and include tags in their clothing, mirrors on the walls (at a child's eye level), or the movement of someone walking by.

Occupational therapists offer various therapies to help children with sensory integration difficulties. Often, timing these therapies with mealtimes improves a child's comfort with food. For more information on this, read chapter 8, "Food Textures and Flavors."

Increase Variety Through Repeated Exposures

Normally, picky eaters go through food jags in which they eat the same foods for several weeks, after which there's a change in the list of acceptable foods. If parents actually count the number of different foods that their child has eaten over three months, they often find that their child has eaten up to thirty different foods. For children with rigid eating, this doesn't happen. Instead it takes considerable effort to teach a child to eat ten to twelve different foods.

Giving kids repeated exposure to problem foods works in the long run, but it is likely to take more time with children diagnosed with autism or sensory aversions. Instead of ten exposures it could require twenty or more. One mother remarked that it often feels like fifty or five hundred.

Don't expect that by trying an endless variety of new foods, you'll discover a food that your child will eat. Usually a systematic introduction of new foods works best. To encourage children to eat more fruit, focus on a single fruit. Instead of offering bananas one day and grapes the next, offer grapes every day. Often children are more open to trying familiar foods that they have learned to touch and smell and have watched others eat.

Consider Food Textures

According to a survey on autistic children done through the University of Louisville, parents cited food texture as the most common reason why a child rejected a food. This is often true for other special needs children as well. When it comes to changing food textures there is one general rule: do it *gradually*.

Here's one child's story:

At age two, Aaron still ate only smooth foods. One of the strategies that helped him move on to lumpy and solid foods was to coat everything with mush. The first time he ate bread, his mother coated it with yogurt. Later, she tried bread dipped in gravy. Gradually, the gravy grew lumpier. His mother added well-cooked, mashed vegetables and then small pieces of meat. Two months later, Aaron was eating mushy turkey sandwiches with visible chunks of meat coated with mashed veggies and gravy. To help him accept the new food textures, he was encouraged to use a Nuk brush and move his tongue, lips, and jaw through play.

A year later, three-year-old Aaron was drinking from a cup, using a spoon by himself, and eating mostly beige foods: pancakes, waffles, grilled cheese, bananas, lemon yogurt, and macaroni and cheese. His parents were pleased. Aaron still resisted new foods with an iron will, but at least he was eating table foods and feeding himself.

If a child likes a crunchy food like potato chips, try to substitute healthier crunchy foods like dry cereal. Then move to crunchy waffles or toast. If a child prefers to drink liquids rather than eat solid foods, try water or lower-calorie drinks to increase the child's appetite for solid foods.

Fill in Nutrition Gaps

Children who eat an extremely limited range of foods for a prolonged period of time have a greater risk for having nutrition gaps in their diet. These gaps may or may not include a need for extra calories. Often a multivitamin offers a simple solution. Other solutions include homemade power foods or fortified foods. These are discussed in chapter 6, "How Much Nutrition Is Enough?"

Some parents of autistic children believe that changing their child's diet improves the symptoms of autism. These gluten- or casein-free diets involve taking a child off foods containing wheat or milk. Some also use vitamin or mineral supplements. Karyn Seroussi, the mother of a child with autism, has written a book about her experiences and cofounded the Autism Network for Dietary Intervention (ANDI). Despite the passionate endorsements of many parents, diet interventions to improve autism remain controversial.

Look for Motivators

If a child enjoys music, play music during meals. You'll probably need to experiment. Different types of music may calm or stimulate while others may motivate a reluctant eater into eating. Sometimes therapists play music a child enjoys only as long as the child continues to eat and turn it off when the child stops.

Other motivators include watching others eat. Puppets, parents, and other children make eating look like fun and inspire children to put food into their mouths. Using toys or television to motivate children to eat is more problematic. Normally, I don't recommend it, although there are situations in which it can help as a short-term remedy.

Find Support

Along with the growing number of children who struggle with food have come professional services to meet their needs. These include one-on-one therapy (most often with an occupational or speech therapist) or group feeding sessions that include other children. Some of these are listed in chapter 13, "Special Services, Tests, and Treatments." Parents can also look for support through local early intervention programs or state health agencies.

You can network with other parents who are dealing with feeding-related problems by joining an electronic mailing list. Look under "Children's Health" on Yahoo!'s message board to find other parents or start your own group.

Other Food-Related Issues

GROWTH

A number of special needs conditions are known to affect a child's growth pattern. A young child with Down syndrome can appear to be underweight when her weight and height are plotted on a standard growth chart, when in fact her growth rate is normal if compared to other girls of her age with Down syndrome. Specialized growth charts are available for a number of conditions, including

Achondroplasia
Cerebral palsy
Down syndrome
Low birth weight
Marfan syndrome
Noonan syndrome
Spina bifida
Turner syndrome
Williams syndrome

These specialized charts are helpful but sometimes imperfect. Many are based on studies done with small numbers of children. It's best to use them in conjunction with the standard growth charts.

Genetic predispositions or too few calories are the most common causes of slow growth. But, if neither of these seems likely, your child may be referred to a pediatric endocrinologist.

HIGH-CALORIE NEEDS

There are a number of conditions that increase a child's calorie needs, including heart defects, immature lungs, cancer, burns, cerebral palsy, and prematurity. Of these, the most common is prematurity. Often babies born prematurely feed more slowly and tire easily. They are also at greater risk for medical complications involving the heart or breathing, which further increase the amount of calories they need to consume.

Brianna was born three months premature. A year and a half

later, she remained small for her age. Her mother, who had three older children, was startled by the amount of food Brianna ate. She remarked, "She's always hungry." Her tiny daughter ate constantly and she wondered if she was feeding her too much.

It turned out that Brianna needed 50 percent more calories than other girls her age and size. Brianna also had BPD (bronchopulmonary dysplasia). Her lungs were not completely developed at birth and her lung capacity remained below average. Both conditions increased her calorie needs.

Whenever a child has increased calorie needs, it is best to keep a closer watch on growth. The ultimate goal is to provide enough calories to enable a child to achieve good growth. The exact number of calories needed to accomplish this will vary with a child's age and medical needs.

If your child is premature, read more about the condition. One helpful book is *Preemies: The Essential Guide for Parents of Premature Babies* by D. W. Wechsler, E. T. Paroli, and M. D. Doron (Pocket Books, 2000).

In addition there are Web sites, such as www.prematurity.org and www.prematureinfant.com.

Feeding Tubes

Tube feedings are used for children with functional digestion who are not able to take in enough food or fluid by mouth to meet their nutritional needs. Examples of conditions in which children may need tube feedings include prematurity, swallowing problems, cystic fibrosis, and cerebral palsy.

Many parents dread using feeding tubes as they can appear cold and clinical. While the image of feeding a child through a tube is decidedly high-tech rather than warm and cuddly, the truth is that feeding tubes are very effective for kids who need to gain substantial weight.

Depending on a child's overall medical needs, feeding tubes may be temporary or long-term. They can be placed through the nose for short-term use, or, more permanently, through the abdomen. If your child's feeding tubes are temporary, it is important to plan for the transition back to eating by mouth. Take steps to keep your child's mouth alive by providing sensations in the mouth during the tube feeding, so that she associates these with the satisfaction that comes from satiety.

Tube feedings offer lots of advantages. Generally kids adapt well to them, suffer little pain, and grow amazingly well. For many, the big challenge comes when it's time to move off the tube and begin to eat food by mouth. Generally this journey requires numerous small steps—some of which have nothing to do with food.

The focus, especially at the beginning, is on getting the mouth ready. "Oral readiness" means having the oral-motor skills (muscle strength and coordination) to eat by mouth and a lack of oral aversion. Overcoming oral aversions can be an obstacle: tube-fed kids are often touchy about anything entering their mouths.

A videotape that gives information on how to overcome oral aversions is *The Journey from Tube Feedings Toward Oral Feeding*. It's available online from www.mealtimenotions.com. Specialty companies like New Visions and Mealtime Notions provide helpful, specialized products and services for parents and professionals.

Because each child is unique, the transition from tube feeding to eating by mouth is rarely straightforward. Before professionals can help, they'll need to know such information as

Early feeding history
Why was the tube put in?

Fine- and gross-motor skills
Cognitive skills

Such information gives professionals a base from which to judge the appropriate next step. For one child that may be tongue exercises; for another it may be sitting at the family table and watching others eat. Generally the steps needed to move forward fall into these three areas: oral-motor, sensory, and behavior.

Don't forget, tube feedings are mealtimes too. Many families try to incorporate the social togetherness that takes place during meals. A mother with five children makes one tube feeding each day a special time for her and her son. This makes her son feel special because he has his mother's undivided attention.

From a medical perspective, tube feeding is relatively simple. Yet parents often face unexpected challenges and emotional stress. Being well-informed makes tube feeding easier and provides tips to make the transition from tube to mouth easier. Kids with Tubes is a good resource. They offer newsletters, conferences, and information for parents and caregivers of tube-fed children. Information is available online at www.kidswithtubes.org.

Food at School

Even if you are making progress at home, you'll need to plan for meals that take place while your child attends school. When special needs children participate in education programs that receive federal funding, there are procedures in place that help ensure that their nutrition needs are addressed. Normally, if your child is under the age of three and enrolled in an early intervention program, you can set feeding goals or outcomes on their IFSP (Individual Family Service Plan).

✕ *Early intervention services are available nationwide. Children with medical or developmental risks are eligible for early intervention services. Although available throughout the country, the services vary from state to state. Services range from screening and referral to direct services. The services begin at birth and end sometime before a child begins school. (The exact age varies from state to state.)*

After early intervention, in order for children to have extra support with meals, they need to have a documented disability or chronic medical condition and a written diet prescription, which is signed by a medical authority. Parents of preschool and school-age children with disabilities should document feeding or special diet needs on their IEP (Individual Education Plan). Children who do not require special education services but who have a chronic medical condition that requires a special diet should have a 504 Accommodation Plan. To learn more about these, contact your state health department.

✕ *A 504 Accommodation Plan is a formal document that enables parents to specify the provisions that a child with special needs requires while attending school. These plans are often a collaboration between parents, the student, and the school. Parents need to make a formal request to obtain these services.*

Although the documents change depending on a child's age, they all serve to map out the services each program provides. If you have particular feeding or nutrition goals for your child, be sure that they are documented and that your child's school is aware of them.

Organizations

Whatever the feeding challenge, parents can benefit from seeking support. There are organizations and programs throughout the country that offer information and services. The following is a partial list.

Autism Society of America
7910 Woodmont Ave., Suite 300
Bethesda, MD 20814-3067
800-328-8476
www.autism-society.org

Celiac Sprue Association
P.O. Box 31700
Omaha, NE 68131-0700
877-272-4272
www.csaceliacs.org

Families for Early Autism Treatment (FEAT)
P.O. Box 255722
Sacramento, CA 95865-5722
916-843-1536
www.feat.org

Federation for Children with Special Needs
95 Berkeley St., Suite 104
Boston, MA 02116
617-482-2915
www.fcsn.org

Gluten Intolerance Group of North America
15110 10th Ave. SW, Suite A
Seattle, WA 98166
206-246-6652
www.gluten.net

Human Growth Foundation
997 Glen Cove Ave., Suite 5
Glen Head, NY 11545
800-451-6434
www.hgfound.org

International Foundation for Gastrointestinal Disorders
P.O. Box 170864
Milwaukee, WI 53217-8076
414-964-1799
www.iffgd.org

Kids with Tubes
59 Sweetwater Ave.
Bedford, MA 01730
617-825-6364
www.kidswithtubes.org

MAGIC (Major Aspects of Growth in Children)
6645 W. North Ave.
Oak Park, IL 60302
708-383-0808
www.magicfoundation.org

March of Dimes
Birth Defects Foundation
1275 Mamaroneck Ave.
White Plains, NY 10605
800-221-4602
www.marchofdimes.com

National Down Syndrome Society
666 Broadway
New York, NY 10012
800-221-4602
www.ndss.org

National Organization for Rare Disorders, Inc. (NORD)
P.O. Box 8923
New Fairfield, CT 06812-8923
800-999-6673
www.rarediseases.org

Spina Bifida Association of America
4590 MacArthur Blvd. NW, Suite 250
Washington, DC 20007-4226
800-621-3141
www.sbaa.org

United Cerebral Palsy Association
1660 L St. NW, Suite 700
Washington, DC 20036
800-872-5827
www.ucp.org

If you are a parent of a child with special needs, reach out and network with other parents and share solutions for mealtime challenges. In addition, there are professionals who provide therapy with benefits that spill over and improve feeding. Some of these are listed in the next chapter.

Do
- Network with other parents to get support and information.
- Contact organizations that offer specific information related to your child's needs.
- Consider the potential impact of medical history or other special needs on your child's growth and calorie needs.

Don't
- Assume responsibility for your child's eating problems.
- Delay getting professional help to solve feeding problems.
- Forget to plan for specialized help your child may need to attend school.

Special Services, Tests, and Treatments

Fussy eating habits, though worrisome and hard to live with, do not, in and of themselves, justify intensive medical tests and specialized treatments. Ordinarily, there needs to be something more. Normally a child who needs specialized services around eating has a developmental lag, poor growth, a behavioral issue, or a medical condition. Any of these can transform fussy eating from an everyday dilemma into a health problem.

DEVELOPMENTAL LAG

A two-year-old who still eats pureed baby foods and refuses table foods isn't demonstrating normal eating habits. The question becomes—why?

Sometimes it's simply because caregivers haven't introduced them yet. In instances when family customs don't explain why a child lacks self-feeding skills or does not eat age-appropriate foods, professionals look further. Are there signs of trouble in the child's mouth? Perhaps there's painful tooth decay. Do mouth muscles lack the strength and coordination needed to bite and chew age-appropriate foods? Does the child drink independently from a cup or bottle? How well can he use fingers, spoon, or fork to eat?

The answers to these questions enable professionals to determine whether or not a child has a developmental delay related to eating.

✕ *If eating problems go beyond the normal level of difficulty, look for professional help. Don't assume responsibility for all your child's eating difficulties. Well-intentioned friends and family sometimes give poor advice. If you suspect your child has special needs, don't delay seeking professional help.*

POOR GROWTH

Judging growth according to a child's appearance doesn't work well. A standardized growth chart is a better guide. Get medical advice if your child's growth (plotted on standard growth charts) falls outside the normal range according to

Size—weight for age is below the fifth percentile
Stature—height for age is below the fifth percentile
Rate of growth—has crossed two channels (dropped two standard deviations) on the growth chart

Any of these growth deviations is a flag to look deeper into picky-eating concerns. It is also often the basis for a child's eligibility for special services, such as individual therapy or a feeding-clinic assessment.

✕ *Check your child's growth status by using a standard growth chart. See chapter 2, "Understanding Growth," for examples of growth charts and information on how to read them.*

MEDICAL CONDITIONS

Kids born prematurely, with a low weight at birth, or with other medical complications have a high risk for problems with growth and eating. Some conditions increase calorie needs. Kids with heart or breathing problems may eat a lot but still grow slowly. Neurological conditions can cause low muscle tone in the mouth and face, making it harder to bite and chew and ultimately take in enough calories.

If your child has a medical condition, ask your doctor about possible effects on eating, digestion, or growth.

If your child has a medical diagnosis, look for specialized support. Depending on the diagnosis, you may find a national organization that provides additional information and support.

BEHAVIORAL ISSUES

Behavior problems around eating are hard to ignore and can include mealtime tantrums, intentional vomiting, pouching, throwing food, or pica (eating nonfood items). Often these behaviors start with a biological cause, which may be subtle enough to go unnoticed. Specialists can offer solutions to treat the underlying cause as well as the behavior.

FINDING HELP

If your picky eater has a developmental lag, a problem with growth, a behavioral problem, or a medical problem, talk to your child's doctor about getting specialized help. Ask for advice on whether your child needs a feeding-team assessment. These are typically associated with a hospital and are described in more detail below.

You may also want to research other services that may be available in your area. You may find short-term feeding programs (consisting of three- to twelve-week sessions) offered through a hospital clinic, an early intervention program, or a private therapy program. Such programs may include small feeding groups for children, parent support groups, or individualized therapy. To find out whether any of these programs are offered in your area, contact the closest hospital feeding clinic, the state department for special education, or the local chapter of the American Occupational Therapy Association. Before enrolling in a program, ask questions about

Experience and training of staff

Type of feeding problems they work with

Track record for helping children with similar feeding problems

In addition, you may find a support group online. Yahoo! offers a number of groups under "Children's Health." You can also find links and information on feeding online at www.congenitalheartdefects.com/feeding.html.

Depending on your child's eating problem, you may want to consult with a nutritionist/dietitian, psychologist, or occupational, physical, or speech therapist. Each of these professional groups has local or state chapters. By contacting them, you can find local listings of those in private practice.

Keep in mind that serious feeding problems take time to resolve and sometimes require more intense evaluation. Because feeding is complex, there are "feeding teams" made up of professionals that provide comprehensive evaluations. As a first step in determining whether or not your child needs this type of evaluation, talk to the pediatrician, or use the PEACH survey (see box below), which was written to enable parents to recognize when a child needs professional help with feeding. Some feeding clinics offer their own questionnaires, which reflect the feeding problems they address.

THE PEACH SURVEY

*Parent Eating and Nutrition Assessment for
Children with Special Health Needs*

Agency: _____ Date:_____

Child's name: _____ Date of birth:_____

Address: _____ Phone #:_____

Please circle *YES* or *NO* for each question as it applies to your child.

Does your child have a health problem (do not   YES   NO (1)
include colds or flu)? If YES, what is it? _____

Is your child: Small for age?___Too thin?___   YES   NO (3)
Too heavy?___ (If you check any of the
above, circle YES.)

Does your child have feeding problems?   YES   NO (3)
If YES, what are they?_____

Is your child's appetite a problem?   YES   NO (1)

Is your child on a special diet?   YES   NO (2)
If YES, what type of diet?_____

Does your child take medicine for a health   YES   NO (1)
problem (do not include vitamins, iron, or
fluoride)? If YES, name the medication._____

Does your child use a feeding tube or other special YES   NO (4)
feeding method? If YES, explain:_____

Does your child have food allergies?   YES   NO (1)
If YES, what are they?_____

Circle YES if your child does **not** eat any of   YES   NO (1)
these foods: *(Check all that apply.)* Milk___
Meats___Vegetables___Fruits   *(continued)*

Circle YES if your child has a problem with   YES   NO (3)
(*Check all that apply.*) Sucking___Swallowing___
Chewing___Gagging___

Circle YES, if your child has a problem with   YES   NO (3)
(*Check all that apply.*) Loose stools___
Hard stools___Throwing Up___Spitting Up___

Does your child eat clay, paint chips, dirt, or   YES   NO (2)
anything else that is not food? If YES, what is it?_____

Does your child refuse to eat, throw food, or do   YES   NO (2)
other things that upset your family mealtime?
If YES, explain:_____

For children **over** 12 months (check if it applies   YES   NO (1)
and circle YES): Is your child **not** using a cup?___
Is your child **not** finger-feeding?___

For children **over** 18 months: Does your child   YES   NO (2)
still take most liquids from a bottle?

Circle YES if your child is **not** using a spoon.   YES   NO (2)

Scoring Instructions:
Add the numbers in the parentheses next to the questions to which
you have answered YES. If you answer YES four or more times or if
your score is 4 or above, ask your pediatrician or early intervention
teacher about a feeding team.

SOURCE: Journal of the American Dietetic Association, October 1994.
Copyright © 1994 by Marci Campbell and Kristine Kelsey. Used with permission.

Places to look for the services of a feeding team include children's therapy centers, children's hospitals or medical centers, early intervention programs, school-based special education programs, and neurodevelopment centers.

Feeding Team Evaluations

Feeding-team evaluations typically include a number of health professionals, each one having a specialized focus. When an interdisciplinary team looks at a child's eating, expect any combination of the following specialists:

Clinical nutritionist/dietitian   *Doctors:*
Nurse   Developmental pediatrician
Occupational therapist   Gastroenterologist
Physical therapist   Psychologist
Social worker   Radiologist
Speech-language pathologist

Exactly what happens in these evaluations varies, but since they all share a common goal of evaluating eating problems, they tend to perform similar activities. The following will give you an idea of what you might expect:

- Observation of the child eating. Sometimes parents are asked to bring food and feed the child as part of the evaluation. Or parents are asked to videotape their child eating at home and bring the tape.
- Assessment of the child's nutrition and growth. Parents complete a food diary listing the foods a child eats. This may be requested in advance or could be part of the evaluation session.
- Looking at the child's position and feeding skills. Professionals compare a child's feeding skills against established norms. Standardized tests are used to rate oral-motor, fine-motor, and gross-motor skills according to age. The results are used as the basis for therapy, with the goal of helping the child gain needed skills.

WHAT DO THEY DO?

Understanding the roles of feeding-team professionals

Clinical nutritionist/dietitian evaluates whether the food a child eats meets calorie and nutrient needs.

Nurse often does weight and height checks and may provide follow-up services in the home.

Occupational therapist looks at a child's fine-motor skills for self-feeding, and in some instances will also evaluate oral-motor skills.

Physical therapist looks at a child's gross-motor skills, and is likely to help with positioning, self-help suggestions, and adaptive equipment.

Social worker may provide supportive counseling, or help co-ordinate community services.

Speech-language pathologist will evaluate the child's oral motor skills and communication skills that may coincide with or contribute to feeding problems. In some instances will collaborate with the radiologist in assessing a child's swallowing.

DOCTORS:

Developmental pediatrician may order routine tests to rule out biological problems or refer the child to a medical specialist.

Gastroenterologist may treat reflux or motility problems that affect feeding.

Psychologist may provide cognitive and developmental evaluation, or work to improve parent-child interactions and reduce stress around feeding.

Radiologist can help characterize swallowing problems.

- If appropriate, other tests may be ordered, such as a barium swallow to explore the effectiveness of swallowing.
- A report may be written up that parents can use as a basis for outside services, such as speech therapy to work on oral-motor

skills, physical therapy to work on better positions for eating, or occupational therapy to work on sensory issues or fine-motor skills.

In many instances, feeding teams provide limited ongoing services. A child who needs follow-up may join a community-based program or return to the medical center for individual therapy or doctor appointments. The written report that feeding teams provide might give recommendations, such as to

- Increase calories by following a recommended schedule for meals and snacks, and using specific high-calorie foods or supplements.
- Modify food textures and consistencies.
- Provide oral-motor activities to strengthen small muscles in the mouth.
- Prepare a child for food with sensory activities, such as using a Nuk brush to stimulate the mouth.
- Improve a child's position to make eating easier or more comfortable.
- Monitor a child's growth with regular weight and height measurements.
- Request additional diagnostic tests.

Tests

PHYSIOLOGY TESTS
Does your child choke, gag, have a history of pneumonia, or have trouble eating table foods? If so, a doctor or feeding specialist may recommend one of the tests below. These tests focus on function and anatomy—they look at the pathway and mechanics of how food travels from the mouth and into the stomach.

- **Upper GI (Gastrointestinal) X-ray** This test goes by different names, including barium swallow, videofluoroscopy (VFS), oral-pharyngeal motility study, cookie swallow, or rehabilitation swallow. There are variations in how the test is conducted. A modified barium swallow is often specified by speech therapists because it is structured to analyze the early phase of swallowing that begins in the mouth.

  For the test, a child is given different foods (containing barium) to swallow, and each one is videotaped. The test is essentially an X-ray movie showing what happens when food is swallowed. The trained eye of a specialist (often a radiologist and a speech therapist) detects obstacles to an effective swallow. This test can find hiatal hernia, blockage, and other problems.

  This test does not require anesthesia or medication. It is not painful, but does involve prodding and positioning, which is sometimes upsetting to a young child. Testing often takes place in the X-ray or radiology department of a hospital as an outpatient procedure.

- **Esophageal pH Probe** A sensor attached to a thin plastic tube is inserted through the nose into the lower part of the esophagus, just above the entrance to the stomach. When stomach acid moves back up into the esophagus the probe detects and records the change in pH. This test confirms acid reflux, but it does not detect whether or not it has caused inflammation or nonacid reflux.

  Normally the probe is left in place for twenty-four hours. Although the recording device may be portable, keeping a child comfortable for the time needed to complete the test can be challenging.

- **Fiberoptic Endoscopic Evaluation of Swallowing (FEES)** This is a relatively new technique for use with children. A small tube with a tiny video camera at the end is slipped through the nose, allowing direct visualization of the oral cavity, nasopharynx, pharynx, and larynx. Because of the technical simplicity of this test, a therapist rather than a physician may perform it.

This test does not require anesthesia or medication. However, toddlers are likely to resist having a tube inserted through the nose. The need for cooperation is a potential problem for using this test with a younger child.

When a child has long-term diarrhea and poor growth, these tests may be recommended:

- **Stool Analysis** The analysis of a stool sample provides evidence for a range of digestive problems, including infections and inflammation.
- **Sweat Chloride Test** This is a specialized test used to confirm cystic fibrosis. A current stimulates the sweat glands and the sweat is analyzed for chloride.

FOOD ALLERGY TESTS

If a food allergy is suspected, your child may have one of the tests listed below. Keep in mind that these are screening tests, best at predicting severe food reactions. For mild or delayed reactions they are less reliable. It is not unusual to test allergic to a food and yet have no reaction when that food is eaten. To fully understand the results of these tests you'll need the advice of a specialist.

- **Skin Test** A diluted amount of the food extract is placed on the skin, the skin is pricked, and the food is allowed to penetrate for about twenty minutes. A small bump appears if there is a reaction. The test is relatively painless and provides quick results. It is more reliable (95 percent) when predicting there is no allergic reaction. The test has a high false-positive rate. As a result, a positive skin test alone does not guarantee that a food reaction will occur.

- **RAST Blood Test** In some cases, this test is used instead of the skin test, especially when a child has eczema, is taking medications, or is at risk for a severe reaction. It measures the presence of specific IgE antibodies to a food allergen. And, as with the skin test, a negative result is more reliable than a positive result. Expect to wait at least one or two weeks for the results.
- **Elimination Diets** These diets eliminate potential problem foods to see if the allergy symptoms go away. There are three types of elimination diets:
  1. Only the food or foods suspected of causing the allergy are avoided; other foods can be eaten. This is the easiest to follow.
  2. Most foods are avoided. A list of "allowed foods" is provided, which lists a small number of low-risk foods. These are the only ones that may be eaten.
  3. A special amino-acid base formula is the only food allowed. This works best for babies but is difficult for older children, partly because kids don't like the taste of these formulas.

This is not a comprehensive list of tests. Any number of other tests may be ordered, including blood tests for lead or iron anemia, growth hormone, and others. A child's medical history determines which tests will be most helpful.

Treatments

MEDICATIONS

Medications that magically solve the problem of fussy eating are, to my knowledge, nonexistent. Although I have seen families use potions and folk remedies, the only medication typically prescribed by a doctor to stimulate appetite is Periactin, which is an antihistamine. Although it sometimes helps, it is not a miracle cure for fussy eating.

On the other hand, many medications affect digestion or appetite as a side effect. The table on page 277 shows potential side effects. Keep in mind that not all children will experience these side effects.

- **Feeding Tubes**

  When a young child is severely underweight, feeding tubes offer a practical solution. Feeding tubes make it easier to give a child extra calories. From a medical perspective, it offers an effective, low-risk solution. Yet many parents struggle with the initial decision and with the day-to-day reality of tube feeding.

  Kids with Tubes is an organization that offers support and information for parents and caregivers of tube-fed children. Information is available online at www.kidswithtubes.org.

  The main benefit of feeding tubes is that they help children to grow. But they do require extra care, such as good hygiene around the insertion site to prevent infection. There is also the risk of kids pulling them out. Lastly, the transition off tube feedings can be stressful. Some of this can be minimized with planning.

- **Fundoplication**

  If a child vomits too much or too often, this surgery offers a solution. Basically, the top portion of the stomach is wrapped more tightly at the base of the esophagus. This is major surgery and is not without risk. However, it may be the best option for a child with severe symptoms for which other treatments have not worked.

POSSIBLE MEDICATION SIDE EFFECTS

MEDICATION	Appetite Loss	Nausea	Vomiting	Diarrhea
Antibiotics				
Amoxicillin	–	+/–	+/–	+
Erythromycin	–	+/–	+	+/–
Acid Reducers				
Metoclopramide (Reglan)	–	+	–	+
Ranitidine (Zantac)	–	+	+	+
Omeprazole (Prilosec)	–	+/–	–	+
Antiseizure				
Carbamazepine	+	+	+	+
Phenobarbital	–	+/–	+/–	–
Phenytoin (Dilantin)	+/–	+	+	–
Anti-ADHD				
Adderall	+	+/–	–	+/–
Atomoxetine	+	+	+	+/–
Methylphenidate (Ritalin)	+	+/–	–	–
Cardiac				
Digoxin	+	+	+	+
Furosemide (Lasix)	+/–	+/–	+/–	+/–
Spironolactone	+/–	+	+	+
Antihypertension				
Clonidine	+/–	+	+	–
Respiratory				
Albuterol inhaler	+/–	+	+	+/–
Beclomethasone	–	+/–	+/–	–
Prednisone	–	+/–	+/–	–

KEY: – rare, +/– occasional (5 percent or more reported), + common (20 percent or more reported)

SOURCE: *Food Medication Interactions*, Zaneta Pronsky, 2004.

If you suspect your child needs specialized help around feeding, don't delay getting services. There are a growing number of programs and services available.

Do
- Consider whether growth, medical conditions, behavior, or developmental needs affect your child's eating.
- Check out the side effects of medications your child takes regularly that may affect eating.
- Seek recommendations from other parents. The quality and range of services vary.

Don't
- Delay finding help for your child. One feeding clinic reported that the average age of the children being referred was thirty-three months.
- Expect that any one service or treatment will instantly solve your child's eating or growth problems. Because of their complex nature, resolving these problems often requires both the right approach and plenty of time.

CLOSING THOUGHTS

In 2005, the U.S. Department of Agriculture updated the food pyramid, the official guide for healthy eating. A few months after releasing written guidelines, the USDA launched an interactive version on the Web. The response was extraordinary. On the first day, an estimated 5.4 million people per hour logged on, overwhelming the site's capacity and, more significantly, demonstrating that millions of Americans want guidance on how to eat better.

These days, the big concern for most Americans is obesity, which on the surface appears unrelated to picky eating. But in fact, the two represent opposite sides of the same coin. The ability to self-regulate calories is the crucial link to health outcome. Both over- and undereating cause problems. More than ever, knowing how much or how little to eat is an important life skill, one that children need encouragement to develop.

Young children are completely dependent on adults to provide their nourishment, and loving parents are usually eager to provide the best. But feeding a young child involves much more than providing food. In order for feeding experiences to go smoothly, a child's maturity, physical needs, and personality must be taken into account. In addition, young children need help to master self-feeding, try new foods, and overcome possible obstacles such as allergies or aversions. All present challenges, which complicate eating and potentially lead to stressful food experiences for children and their parents.

Children who don't learn to self-feed or enjoy new foods, or who have other problems with eating, may be "problem feeders" or "resistant eaters." In such cases, parents may worry that they are somehow to blame when, in fact, their child just needs extra help. Professionals are trained to look at feeding problems more closely and offer therapies designed to expand the number of foods a child can eat and enjoy.

But most picky eaters do not have feeding problems that require professional intervention. According to researchers, the majority of complaints about picky eating coincide with the time that a child's growth slows down and he begins to establish independence. Concerned parents who try to help picky eaters make better food choices at this stage often find that their children don't appreciate parental food guidance. Even one-year-olds may insist on eating as they please. All the same, many parents persist. They try to prod their child to eat and make demands like "Just two more bites."

Loving parents are justified in helping their child make better food choices. But in light of the growing number of eating problems among Americans, the question is, does it work?

There's quite a bit of research on the social dynamics around food and whether this influences the ability to accurately self-regulate calories. This is not an entirely new topic for researchers. In 1928, Dr. Clara M. Davis published a landmark study that looked at the eating patterns of young children and babies. She specifically looked at the effects of how food was presented to children.

The children were given three to four meals a day with nothing but water offered between meals. At each meal, a tray with eleven to fourteen different foods was placed in front of each child. Although they were given help if needed, the children ate freely without either encouragement or coercion.

Not surprisingly, there were times when children ate odd combinations or large amounts of one food. One day, one of the boys ate ten eggs! But overall the children chose a reasonably balanced diet. Many of the foods kids liked then are still popular. Almost all the kids liked fruit, and for many of the children, it made up half of their daily calories. Overall, the most popular foods were meats, potatoes, carrots, peas, eggs, milk, bananas, and orange juice. The least popular foods were spinach, lettuce, turnips, and barley. During the study, the children had no digestive upsets; they enjoyed eating, grew well and were healthy.

Since 1928, other researchers have continued to confirm that children eat best when they are allowed to control their own eating. Of course, this doesn't mean letting young children eat junk foods. Normally parents control the supply of foods for young children and this is the time to make a point to offer healthy foods in a pleasant manner. Which foods a child eats or doesn't eat is not the only issue. It's also important that young children practice making their own food choices with family support and encouragement.

All too soon kids will begin making their own food choices without parental help or supervision. One of the best things a parent can do is to prepare them. While a plea to a child for "just two more bites," is understandable, with some thought and deeper understanding, parents can find more effective solutions.

BIBLIOGRAPHY

Introduction

Tucker, M. E., "Serious feeding disorders call for intensive therapy." *Pediatric News* 3 (2002): 35.

Winters, N. C. "Feeding problems in infancy and early childhood." *Primary Psychiatry* 10 (2003): 30–34.

Chapter 1: Solving the Puzzle of Picky Eating

Hawdon, J., N. Beauregard, J. Slattery, and G. Kennedy. "Identification of neonates at risk of developing feeding problems in infancy." *Developmental Medicine and Child Neurology* 42 (2000): 235–39.

Hearn, M., T. Baranowski, J. Baranowski, et al. "Environmental influences on dietary behavior among children: availability and accessibility of fruits and vegetables enable consumption." *Journal of Health Education* 29 (1998): 26–32.

Jahns, L., A. M. Siega-Riz, and B. M. Popkin. "The increasing prevalence of snacking among U.S. children from 1977–1996." *Journal of Pediatrics* 138 (2001): 493–98.

Kedesdy, J. H., and K. S. Budd. *Childhood Feeding Disorders.* Baltimore: Paul H. Brookes Publishing Co., 1998.

Manikam, R., and J. Perman, "Pediatric Feeding Disorders." *Journal of Clinical Gastroenterology* 30 (2000): 1688–1703.

Rozin, P., and D. Schiller. "The nature and acquisition of a preference for chili peppers in humans." *Motive and Emotion* 4 (1980): 77–101.

Stockmyer, C. "Remember when mom wanted you home for dinner?" *Nutrition Reviews* 59 (2001): 57–60.

Sullivan, S. A., and L. L. Birch. "Pass the sugar, pass the salt, experience dictates preference." *Developmental Clinical Psychology and Psychiatry* 26 (1990): 546–51.

Walton, C. "When picky becomes a problem." *Detroit Free Press,* June 11, 2002.

Chapter 2: Understanding Growth

Kuczmarksi, R., W. Dietz, R. Berhane, and H. Cloud. "The New Growth Charts: Who, What, When and How?" Videoconference sponsored by University of Alabama and U.S. Maternal and Child Health Bureau, May 25, 1999.

Stephenson, L. S., M. C. Latham, and A. Jansen. *A Comparison of Growth Standards: Similarities Between NCHS, Harvard, Denver and Privileged African Children and Differences with Kenyan Rural Children.* New York, Cornell International Nutrition Monograph Series, no. 12, 1983.

U.S. Department of Health and Human Services, National Center for Health Statistics. "CDC Growth Charts." *Advance Data,* no. 314, June 8, 2000 (revised), 1–7.

Walker, A., and K. Hendricks. *Manual of Pediatric Nutrition.* W.B. Saunders Co., 1985.

Chapter 3: Feeding Skills

Illingworth, R. S., and J. Lister. "The critical or sensitive period with special reference to certain feeding problems in infants and children." *Journal of Pediatrics* 65 (1964): 839.

Klein, M. D., and T. Delaney. *Feeding and Nutrition for the Child with Special Needs.* San Antonio: Therapy Skill Builders, 1994.

Morris, S. E. *The Normal Acquisition of Oral Feeding Skills: Implications for Assessment and Treatment.* Santa Barbara: Therapeutic Media Inc., 1982.

Rogers, S. J., C. M. Donovan, D. D'Eugenio, S. Brown, E. W. Lynch, M. Moersch, and D. S. Schafer. Developmental Programming for Infants and Young Children, vol. 2, Early Intervention Developmental Profile.

Chapter 4: Fussy Babies

Celedon, J. C., A. A. Litonjua, L. Ryan, S. T. Weiss, and D. R. Gold. "Bottle feeding in the bed or crib before sleep time and wheezing in early childhood." *Pediatrics* 6 (2002): e77

Chatoor, I., R. Hirsh, and M. Persinger. "Facilitating internal regulation of eating: a treatment model for infantile anorexia." *Infants and Young Children* 9 (1997): 12–22.

Gerrish, C. J., and J. A. Mennella. "Flavor variety enhances food acceptance in formula-fed infants." *American Journal of Clinical Nutrition* 73 (2001): 1080–85.

Mennella, J. A. "Early flavor experiences: when do they start?" *Nutrition Today,* September/October 1994.

Mennella, J. A., and G. K. Beauchamp. "Maternal diet alters the sensory qualities of human milk and the nursling's behavior." *Pediatrics* (1991): 737–44.

Mennella, J. A., C. J. Jagnow, and G. K. Beauchamp. "Prenatal and postnatal flavor learning by human infants." *Pediatrics* 6 (2001): 107.

Pitman, T. "Is it gas?" *Today's Parent,* December/January 2005.

Skinner, J. D., B. R. Carruth, B. Bounds, P. Ziegler, and K. Reidy. "Do food-related experiences in the first two years of life predict dietary variety in school-aged children?" *Journal of Nutrition Education and Behavior* 34 (2002): 310–15.

Sullivan, S. A., and L. L. Birch. "Infant dietary experience and acceptance of solid foods." *Pediatrics* 93 (1994): 271–77.

Chapter 5: Fussy Toddlers and Preschoolers

"Brain Development: Frequently Asked Questions. www.zerotothree. org/brainwonders/FAQ-body.html.

Chatoor, I., R. Hirsch, and M. Persinger. "Facilitating internal regulation of eating: a treatment model for infantile anorexia." *Infants and Young Children* 9 (1997): 12.

Foy, T., D. Czyzewski, S. Philips, B. Ligon, J. Baldwin, and W. Klish. "Treatment of severe feeding refusal in infants and toddlers." *Infants and Young Children* 9 (1997): 26. Aspen Publishers, Inc.

"How Nutrition Affects Cognition: Implications for Feeding Infants and Children." 29th Annual Current Issues in Nutrition, satellite videoconference, Iowa State University, April 27, 2000.

Johnson, S. L. "Improving preschoolers' self-regulation of energy intake." *Pediatrics* 106 (December 2000): 1429.

Report of informal meeting to review and develop indicators for complementary feeding. Washington, D.C., World Health Organization, 2002.

Wolf, R. P., and C. J. Lierman. "Management of behavioral feeding problems in young children." *Infants and Young Children* 7 (1994): 14.

Worthington-Roberts, B. S., and S. Williams. *Nutrition Throughout the Life Cycle.* New York: McGraw-Hill, 2000.

Chapter 6: How Much Nutrition Is Enough?

Beal, V. A. *Nutrition in the Life Span.* John Wiley, 1980.

Davis, C. M. "Self-selection of diets by newly weaned infants: an experimental study." *American Journal of Diseases of Children* 36 (1928): 651–79.

"Dietary Reference Intakes." Institute of Medicine of the National Academies. www.iom.edu.

Kleinman, R. E., *Pediatric Handbook,* 5th ed. American Academy of Pediatrics, 2004.

Roberts, L. R. *Nutrition Work with Children.* University of Chicago Press, 1936.

Shils, M. E., J. A. Olson, M. Shike, A. C. Ross (eds.). *Modern Nutrition in Health and Disease,* 9th ed. Philadelphia: Lippincott, Williams and Wilkins, 1999.

Chapter 7: Making Food Desirable

Beauchamp, G. K. "The Development in Taste in Infancy." In J. T. Ond, L. J. Filer, G. A. Leveille, A. Thompson, and W. B. Weil (eds.). *Infant and Early Childhood Feeding.* New York: Academic Press, 1981.

Beauchamp, G. K., and O. Maller. "The Development of Flavor Preferences in Humans: a Review." In M. R. Kare and O. Maller (eds.). *The Chemical Senses and Nutrition.* Academic Press, 1977.

Blumenthal, M., et al. (eds.), S. Klein, and R. S. Rister (trans.). *The Complete German E Monographs: Therapeutic Guide to Herbal Medicines.* American Botanical Council and Integrative Medicine, 1998.

Branen L., J. Fletcher, and L. Hilbert. "Snack consumption and waste by preschool children served 'cute' versus regular snacks." *Journal of Nutrition Education and Behavior* 34 (2002): 279.

Howard, R. (ed.), and H. Winter. *Nutrition and Feeding of Infants and Toddlers.* Boston: Little, Brown, and Company, 1984.

Leveille, G. A., M. E. Zabik, and K. J. Morgan. *Nutrients in Food.* Cambridge, MA: The Nutrition Guild, 1983.

Chapter 8: Food Textures and Flavors

Frick, S., R. Frick, P. Oetter, and E. Richter. *Out of the Mouths of Babes.* Hugo, Minnesota: PDP Press, Inc., 1996.

Gisel, E. G. "Effect of food texture on the development of chewing of children between six months and two years of age." *Developmental Medicine and Child Neurology* 33 (1991): 69–79.

Haron, M. "Nutrition and Sensory Integration." *OTA Newsline* (Occupational Therapy Associates; Watertown, MA), fall 2001.

Liem, D. G., and J. Mennella. "Heightened sour preferences during childhood." *Chemical Senses* 28 (2003): 173–80.

McGowan, K. "The science of scrumptious." *Psychology Today,* September/October 2003.

Toomey, K., E. S. Ross, and S. T. Massey, "Picky Eaters vs. Problem Feeders: The SOS Approach to Feeding." Conference sponsored by Education Resources Inc., August 11, 2005.

Chapter 9: Family Influences

Agras, S., L. Hammer, and F. McNicolas. "A prospective study of the influence of eating-disordered mothers on their children." *International Journal of Eating Disorders* 3 (1999): 253–62.

Birch, L. L., and J. O. Fisher. "Development of eating behaviors among children and adolescents." *Pediatrics* 101 (1998): 539–49.

Birch, L. L., J. O. Fisher, and K. K. Davison. "Learning to overeat: maternal use of restrictive feeding practices promotes girls' eating in the absence of hunger." *American Journal of Clinical Nutrition* 78 (2003): 215–20.

Boyton-Jarrett, R. "Impact of television viewing patterns on fruit and vegetable consumption on adolescents." *Pediatrics* (2003).

Brown, R., and J. Ogden. "Children's eating attitudes and behavior: a study of the modelling and control theory of parental influence." *Health Education Research* 19 (2004): 261–71.

Butte, N., K. Cobb, J. Dwyer, L. Graney, W. Heird, and K. Richard. "The start healthy feeding guidelines of infants and toddlers". *Journal of the American Dietetic Association* 104 (2004): 442–54.

Carruth, B., P. Ziegler, H. Gordon, and S. Barr. "Prevalence of picky eaters among infants and toddlers and their caregivers decisions about offering a new food." *Journal of the American Dietetic Association* 104 (2004): S57–S64.

Fisher, J. O., and L. L. Birch. "Restricting access to foods and children's eating." *Appetite* 32 (1999): 405–19.

Gillman, M. W., and Rifas. "Family dinner and diet quality among older children and adolescents." *Archives of Family Medicine,* vol. 9, no. 3, March 2000.

Kane, C. "Television and Movie Characters Sell Children Snacks." *New York Times,* December 8, 2003, C7.

Nestle, M. *Food Politics: How the Food Industry Influences Nutrition and Health.* University of California Press, 2002.

Pereira, J., and A. Warren. "Call for Tighter Restrictions on Kids' Ads, As Focus Turns to Possible TV-Obesity Link." *Wall Street Journal,* March 15, 2004, B1.

Schlosser, Eric. *Fast Food Nation.* HarperCollins, 2001.

Story, M., and S. French. "Food advertising and marketing directed at children." *The International Journal of Behavioral Nutrition and Physical Activity,* Dec. 9, 2004.

———. "Top 200 Megabrands." *Advertising Age,* October 11, 2004, S8–10.

Chapter 10: Mealtime Do's and Don'ts

Coon, K. A., J. Goldberg, B. L. Rogers, and K. L. Tucker. "Relationships between use of television during meals and children's food consumption patterns." *Pediatrics* 107 (2001): e7.

Fisher, J. O., and L. L. Birch. "Restricting access to palatable foods affects children's behavioral response, food selection, and intake." *American Journal of Clinical Nutrition* 69 (1999): 1264.

Gallo, A. "Food Advertising in the United States." *America's Eating Habits: Changes and Consequences.* Washington, D.C., Economic Research Service, U.S. Department of Agriculture, 1999.

Wolff, R. P., and C. J. Lierman. "Management of behavioral feeding problems in young children." *Infants and Young Children* 79 (1994): 14–23.

Chapter 11: Food Allergies and Digestion Problems

Hine, C. L., R. J. Parker and W. Burks. "Food allergies in children affect nutrient intake and growth." *Journal of the American Dietetic Association* 11 (2002): 1648–51.

Locke, G. R., J. H. Pemberton, and S. F. Phillips. "AGA technical review on constipation." *Gastroenterology* 119 (2000): 1766–78.

Markowitz, J. E., and C. A. Liacouras. "Eosinophilic esophagitis." *Gastroenterology Clinics of North America* 32 (2003): 949–66.

Seidman, E. G., and S. Singer. "Therapeutic modalities for cow's milk allergy." *Annals of Allergy, Asthma, and Immunology* 90 (2003): 104–11.

Sicherer, S. H. "Clinical aspects of gastrointestinal food allergy in childhood." *Pediatrics* 111 (2003): 1609–15.

Chapter 12: Feeding a Child with Special Needs

Foy, T., D. Czyzewski, S. Phillips, B. Ligon, and W. Klish. "Treatment of severe feeding refusal in infants and toddlers." *Infants and Young Children* 9 (1997): 26–35.

Growth References, 2nd ed. Clinton, SC: Greenwood Genetic Center, 1997.

Issacs, J. S., J. Cialone, J. Horsley, M. Holland, P., and M. Nardella. *Children with Special Health Care Needs: A Community Pocket Guide.* The American Dietetic Association, 1997.

Krick P., J. Murphy-Miller, S. Zeger, and E. Wright. "Pattern of growth in children with cerebral palsy." *Journal of the American Dietetic Association* 96 (1996): 680–85.

Medlen, J. G. *The Down Syndrome Nutrition Handbook.* Bethesda, MD: Woodbine House, 2002.

Nardella, M., L. Campo, and B. Ogata (eds.). *Nutrition Interventions for Children with Special Health Care Needs.* Washington State Department of Health, 2nd ed., May 2002.

Ohio Neonatal Nutritionists: Nutritional Care for High Risk Newborns. Philadelphia: George F. Stickney Co., 1994.

Quinn, H. P., and K. Levine. "Nutrition Concerns for Children with Pervasive Developmental Disorder/Autism." Center on Human Development and Disability, University of Washington, *Nutrition Focus* (1995), 10:5.

U.S. Department of Education, *Twenty-first Annual Report to Congress on the Implementation of the Individuals with Disabilities Education Act.* Washington, DC, 1999.

Williams, G. P., N. Dalrymple, and J. Neal. "Eating habits of children with autism." *Pediatric Nursing* 26 (2000): 259.

Chapter 13: Special Services, Tests, and Treatments

Kelsey, K., and M. Campbell. "PEACH survey." *Journal of the American Dietetic Association* 92 (1994): 1439.

Lindblom, M., "Therapy Aims to Help Youngsters Overcome the Fear of Food." *Seattle Times,* February 7, 2000.

Pronsky, Z. *Food Medication Interactions,* 13th ed., 2004.

Strickland, E. *Nutrition Therapy: For Children with Autism Spectrum Disorder.* Nashville, TN: Cross Country Education, Inc., 2005.

INDEX

A

Advertising, food-related, 177–80, 189

Allergies
versus adverse food reactions, 210–211
allergy-free vitamins, 113
buying special foods, 220
cookbook resources, 220–21
to eggs, 213–14, 217
genetic dispositions, 211
helping kids cope with, 221–22
to milk, 212–13, 217
to multiple foods, 219
outgrowing, 210, 218
to peanuts, 210, 214–15, 218
physical symptoms, 210–12
to pollen, 222
psychological reactions to, 212, 219–20
reading food labels, 216–18
to soy products, 215–16
testing for, 218, 274–75
to wheat, 215

Anemia, 98, 99, 104

Appetite, 8, 31, 60, 189, 198, 256

Asthma, 113

Autism, 7, 147, 249–50, 253

B

Babies
bottle-fed, 35–36, 67–68, 74–75
breast-fed, 35–36, 68, 74–75
developmental influences, 6–7, 35–38
feeding challenges, 65–73
feeding guidelines, 59–65, 177
ideal new food stages, 35–38

Behavioral issues, 81–83, 190–91, 242–43, 266

Biological influences, 8–9

Body Mass Index (BMI), 29

Books, food-related, for kids, 138–42

Books, on allergy-free cooking, 220–21

Bottle-fed babies, 35–36, 67–68, 74–75

Breast-fed babies, 35–36, 68, 74–75

Breast milk, thickening, 160

Bribes, 10–11, 189–90

C

Calcium, 94–95

Calories, 26, 31, 70, 104–6, 109, 187, 255–56, 266

Carrot juice study, 74

Casein, 213

Celiac disease, 8, 236

Cereals, fiber-rich, 226

Chewing, 37–38, 145

Choking, 145

Colic, 69

Color of food, 146–47

Congestion, 222

Constipation, 223–31

Constitutional Growth Delay (CGD), 31

Control issues, 143, 190, 243

Cooking activities, 127–29, 201

Cup, transition to, 36

Cup design features, 130–33

D

Decongestants, 222

Dehydration, 158, 229, 241

Developmental influences, 5–7

Diapers, 233

Diarrhea, 232–37

Digestive problems, 8, 68–69

Dining tables, 198–199

Dishes, 137

Distractions, mealtime, 188–89, 251

Down syndrome, 247, 254–55

Drooling, 48–49

E

Early Intervention, 220, 259

Eating disorders, adult, 15–16, 171–72, 191

Eating utensils and gear, 129–38

Egg allergies, 213–14, 217